LACTATE LIFT-OFF

LACTATE
LIFT-OFF

BY OWEN ANDERSON, PH. D.

SSS Publishing Inc.
Lansing, MI

First Edition

The text of this book is composed in 10/12 Palatino.
Printing by Ledges' Printing Inc.
Cover design by Mike Dyson
Book design by Jim Bledsoe
Exercises by Walt Reynolds, C.S.C.S.

Library of Congress Cataloging-in-Publication Data
Anderson, Owen.
Lactate Lift-Off / by Owen Anderson, Ph. D.

Library of Congress Catalog Card Number 98-96158

ISBN 0-9663726-0-3

SSS Publishing, Inc., 1433 Sunnyside Ave, Lansing, MI 48910
USA

1 2 3 4 5 6 7 8 9 0

For Teressa,
who has given me the
ultimate gift of life itself

And for my parents,
who have always been there

LACTATE LIFT-OFF

CHAPTER 1

AN LT STORY

When Marc Rogers traveled to St. Louis in July, 1984 to begin his post-graduate research in exercise physiology at Washington University, he also commenced training for the St. Louis Marathon, which was scheduled for the following November. Before getting into his hard-core marathon preparations, Marc underwent an exercise test in the St. Louis lab and learned that his maximal aerobic capacity (VO_2max) was 70 ml/kg/min, while his lactate-threshold (LT) running velocity was reached at 78 percent of VO_2max, or at 54.6 ml/kg/min.

Marc proceeded to train very aggressively, combining high-intensity work with high mileage (about 80 miles per week), and was re-tested in early November. Despite the heavy-duty training, Marc's VO_2max had moved upward by nary a milliliter of oxygen, clinging stubbornly to the same 70-ml mark of mid-summer. Fortunately, though, Marc's LT had "gone through the roof," climbing from 78 to a lusty 90 percent of VO2max (or 63 ml/kg/min). And yes - Marc won the St. Louis Marathon that fall, primarily because of his huge advance in LT.

You may not win a major marathon, as Marc did, but you, too, can make major improvements in your LT, regardless of your current ability level. The good news is that your LT upgrade will make you a dramatically fitter person and - if you like to enter races - a considerably more competitive athlete. That's because LT is the best-possible predictor of physical performance in all activities which last for two minutes or more. It is better than VO2max, and it's also superior to athletic economy (efficiency of movement), strength, power, flexibility, agility, or any other measure of athletic prowess. If you want to reach your ultimate fitness and performance goals, you must travel along the pathway of LT improvement.

This book tells you *why* LT is such a great predictor of fitness and performance and shows you exactly *how* to improve your LT to the greatest possible extent. If you follow the principles outlined in this book, you will be able to reach goals which previously seemed unattainable. Fortunately, LT improvement is rather straightforward. Although it is often presented as an extremely complex undertaking, LT training does not have to be highly sophisticated or "high-tech". You won't need to actually measure your blood lactate levels when you train, and for most of the workouts (especially if you are a runner), you won't even need to worry about heart rate.

Best of all, LT workouts are for individuals of all ability levels - and all ages. Beginning runners, bikers, and walkers will experience major gains in fitness with just two LT sessions per week. At the other end of the spectrum, elite athletes may be able to make major performance gains *only* by shooting for an LT lift-off. Masters athletes can keep up with younger performers by focusing intently on LT, because - fortunately - LT remains very responsive to training, even beyond the age of 70! While other key physiological variables like VO_2max and economy are stagnating or declining, LT may continue to push upward in older athletes. The bottom line is that LT training is for everyone. It will make a huge difference in what you are able to do!

OWEN ANDERSON

CHAPTER 2

THINGS YOUR MOM FORGOT
TO TELL YOU ABOUT GLYCOLYSIS

To understand what actually happened to Marc Rogers, the St. Louis Marathon winner we mentioned in Chapter One, and to comprehend how you, too, can make major gains in LT and performance, we need to tell a tale about a chemical compound called lactate. The first part of this lactate parable will center around a key physiological process called *glycolysis*. If . you don't like science, or if you find the biochemical interactions explained in this chapter to be rough going, don't worry! You will still be able to understand and carry out the LT workouts described in subsequent chapters, and you'll make huge gains in your fitness and performance.

Glycolysis is such an important process that if your muscles lost their ability to carry it out, you would never be able to run another 5K or marathon, complete a 40-K bike race, or swim competitively at any distance.

15

In fact, without glycolysis you wouldn't be able to ride around the block on your bike or even walk to the corner store in a reasonable amount of time. Glycolysis is actually a series of 10 different chemical reactions (don't worry - we won't ask you to memorize them) which break down glucose, the simple six-carbon sugar which is your body's most important source of carbohydrate fuel, into something called pyruvic acid. This glycolytic conversion of glucose to pyruvic acid quickly produces some of the energy your muscles need for exercise.

However, for endurance athletes the most important aspect of glycolysis is actually what happens *after* the glycolytic reactions take place: The pyruvic acid created during glycolysis can be funneled into a complex series of energy-creating reactions called the Krebs cycle. In addition to "handling" the pyruvic acid produced from glucose, the Krebs cycle also metabolizes fats; overall, it furnishes more than 90 percent of the energy you need to exercise in a sustained manner. Since glycolysis provides your muscles with quick energy and also "jump-starts" the Krebs cycle, it is a paramount player in muscular energy production. In fact, without glycolysis your muscles would grind to a halt after only 10 to 15 seconds of activity; if you were attempting to run, your legs would feel like a pair of pressure-treated wooden fence posts, and your dynamic strides would quickly change to an inchmeal hobble.

Fortunately, glycolysis usually proceeds normally inside your muscle cells without your having to worry about it, and it also tends to "keep pace" with your activity; the faster you run, cycle, ski, swim, or move during any other sustained activity, the "hotter" your glycolysis fires burn. This has a very interesting consequence: Not all of the pyruvic acid produced via glycolysis can be instantaneously shuttled into the Krebs cycle; as it waits to get onboard the "Krebs-cycle train", an enzyme called lactic dehydrogenase can convert some of the pyruvic acid to lactic acid (you knew we would get to lactic acid eventually). If your muscles are at rest or engaged in moderate activity, only a small amount of lactic acid will be formed. However, if you are exercising strenuously, glucose is broken down to pyruvic acid at very high rates, and lots and lots of pyruvic acid may be waiting around in the Krebs-cycle "queue". As a result, unusually large amounts of lactic acid can be formed.

OWEN ANDERSON

CHAPTER 3

THE TRUTH ABOUT LACTIC ACID

So far, you've learned that lactic acid can appear in your muscle cells rather readily: As your muscles carry out the process of glycolysis to obtain valuable energy and jump-start the Krebs cycle, pyruvic acid and lactic acid are naturally formed. If you're an active person, you have probably read some things about lactic acid in other books, as well as in running and fitness magazines. You're probably no stranger to the idea that lactic acid appears in greater amounts when you are moving along quickly. In fact, you probably believe that the "burn" you feel in your leg muscles when you're running fast or pedaling strenuously on your bike is caused by lactic acid - and that the soreness you experience the day after an especially tough workout is produced by the same "troublesome" compound. You may also cling to the idea that lactic acid is a "waste product" formed in your muscles during vigorous exercise, and that lactic acid shows up in your muscles when you "run out" of oxygen, or because you've gone into "oxygen debt." In short, you probably believe that lactic acid is really bad stuff!

Well, it isn't! All of the above statements are untrue: Lactic acid doesn't produce burning sensations, it does not induce soreness, and it's not a form of metabolic "garbage" which must be eliminated from your cells as quickly as possible. In addition, oxygen shortfalls are not required in order to make lactic acid appear in your muscles and blood. The truth is that lactic acid is produced in your body all the time, around the clock, even when you're at rest (remember that it's a natural by-product of the key energy-producing process called glycolysis), and its concentrations can rise rather dramatically whenever you take in a carbohydrate-containing meal. If lactic acid really caused soreness, you would experience muscle pain every time you wolfed down a Power Bar® or a bowl of rice! Fortunately, we're not telling you all this in order to improve your chances of gaining a Ph. D. in cell physiology: We're giving you the straight scoop because an understanding of how lactic acid actually functions in your body can improve your fitness and endurance performances tremendously!

You see, instead of being a dangerous compound which wreaks havoc inside muscle cells, lactic acid (or more accurately, lactate) plays a paramount role in the processing of the carbohydrate you eat, helping to make that carbohydrate more readily available to your tissues. In addition, lactate helps keep your liver and muscles stockpiled with carbohydrate (those are two critically important roles, because the liver relies on carbohydrate to maintain normal blood-sugar levels, and the muscles utilize carbohydrate as a key energy source during sustained activity). Up to 50 percent of the lactate you produce during a very tough workout may be used to synthesize glycogen in your muscles (glycogen is the key storage form of carbohydrate in your body). Far from damaging your tissues or inducing soreness, this glycogen provides you with the energy you need to carry out subsequent high-quality workouts, because the glycogen can be broken down into countless molecules of glucose, which then undergo glycolysis ("Disposal of Lactate during and after Strenuous Exercise in Humans," *Journal of Applied Physiology*, vol. 61(1), pp. 338-343, 1986). *During* exercise, lactate is also an irreplaceable source of immediate energy for muscles and other tissues, so much so that enhancing your ability to "process" lactate can improve your race times rather dramatically. If you're a typical endurance athlete, the "lactate training techniques" outlined in this book should hasten your performances by anywhere from 4 to 20 percent!

As if that weren't enough, many physiologists believe that lactate also helps keep you from getting fat. To understand how that might happen, let's pretend that you have just finished a high-carbohydrate meal. Much of the carbohydrate in that repast enters your bloodstream as glucose - and heads straight for your liver. The liver picks up a truck-load of this glucose - and converts much of it (via glycolysis) to lactate. This lactate is then "released" from the liver into the bloodstream, destined for "all points" around your body.

Why does the liver like to ship out carbohydrate as lactate? Why doesn't it simply keep the carbohydrate packaged as pure glucose? It's actually a great move on the liver's part, because glucose tends to enter body tissues (including the muscles) rather sluggishly. Glucose must be "guided" into tissues by an important hormone called insulin, and the overall process can be compared to the movement of molasses on a cold Michigan day (that's why your blood-sugar levels tend to stay high for a couple of hours after a carbohydrate-rich meal). Lactate, on the other hand, doesn't depend on insulin and can enter muscle and other cells very quickly. Lactate is quick energy for your tissues! It represents a "short-cut" in the process of transferring energy from your plate to your muscles.

This overall process means that blood levels of both glucose and lactate rise after you've had a high-carbohydrate meal. However, lactate levels don't appear to rise as fast as glucose concentrations, primarily because lactate is rapidly removed from the blood once it appears, while glucose is taken away more slowly. As mentioned, by changing some of the absorbed glucose from your collation over to lactate, your liver quickens the "disposal" of blood carbohydrate. A key benefit of this glucose-lactate conversion is that the amount of insulin which pours into the blood from your pancreas decreases (the higher the glucose level, the greater the insulin response). This limiting of insulin production helps to prevent wild upswings in fat formation (one of the "bad" points about insulin is that it coaxes glucose into adipose cells, where it can readily be converted into blubber).

The Lactate Shuttle

Lactate is also the primary player in another extremely important process called the "lactate shuttle". Described by George Brooks and his colleagues at the University of California-Berkeley, the lactate shuttle involves the following chain of events:

(1) Lactate is formed in ample amounts in tissues in which glycogen and glucose are being broken down at high rates (for example, in your leg muscles when you are running, cycling, or swimming at a strenuous pace). As we indicated earlier, pyruvate is actually formed first, but pyruvate can be readily converted to lactate.

(2) The lactate formed from pyruvate can slip quickly and quietly out of cells and into surrounding tissues and the blood. This "lactate escape" in effect enables glycolysis (the conversion of glucose into pyruvate) to keep going at high rates (if pyruvate could not be transformed into dispersible lactate, pyruvate might build up to overly generous levels within muscle cells; this would shut down glycolysis and - of course - thwart energy production). As lactate departs from hard-working muscle cells, it can be "picked up" by nearby muscle cells, or it can enter the bloodstream and be transported

to other muscles and tissues throughout the body.

(3) The muscle cells and tissues receiving the lactate have a couple of choices: (1) They can utilize it as an energy-rich fuel by converting it back to pyruvate and sending it into the Krebs cycle (lactate is a rich source of ATP, the key "energy currency" within cells), or (2) they can use lactate as a building block in the formation of glycogen. Any glycogen created from lactate can simply hang around quietly in cells until energy is needed at a later time.

The lactate shuttle shows us again that lactate is very far from being a "toxin", a "metabolic waste product", or a key inducer of fatigue, as it is often described. Lactate's easy diffusibility prevents glycolysis from shutting down, and its "high-octane" fuel status helps a variety of cells satisfy their immediate energy requirements or else store energy for future use.

CHAPTER 4

WHAT IS THE
LACTATE THRESHOLD?

Our descriptions of lactate's activities help you comprehend that somewhat mysterious phenomenom called the lactate threshold, or LT. When you begin a moderate to difficult workout, lactate levels in your blood initially rise, simply because glycolysis is working away to provide quite a bit of the energy you require. If there were plenty of oxygen around, the pyruvate formed from glycolysis could enter the Krebs cycle and "be broken down all the way" to carbon dioxide and water, releasing a lot of important energy in the process. However, because you've just started your workout and therefore blood and oxygen flow to your muscles is still somewhat minimal (heart rate is just beginning to rise, and capillaries leading into the muscles are not yet in the full-open position), a fair amount of pyruvate will be converted to lactate, and lactate will pile up inside your leg-muscle cells and begin spilling out into the blood. If we measured your blood-lactate levels at this early stage of your workout, we might find surprisingly high concentrations of lactate, even if you were moving along at a pretty modest pace.

If you keep running, cycling, or swimming at a temperate pace, your blood lactate will quickly simmer down, however. As heart rate increases and capillaries dilate, oxygen will pour into your muscle cells, pyruvate and lactate will be oxidized for energy, and the spillover process will abate. Your blood-lactate levels will drop a bit and then hold steady, which simply means that the entry and exit rates of lactate into and out of your blood are equal (some lactate will no doubt continue to be spilled into the blood, but your muscles and other tissues will remove this "spillage" approximately as fast as it appears).

And lactate levels may hold steady, even as you gradually increase the intensity of your workout As long as you're not going too fast, e. g., as long as enough oxygen is moving into your muscle cells to "take care" of the pyruvate produced by glycolysis and thus control the lactate spillage, your blood lactate will appear to be as calm as a small Iowa farm pond on a windless day.

However, once you get up to a point (actually to a speed) at which glycolysis is tearing along so fast that your leg muscles have problems converting most of the pyruvate and lactate being formed to carbon dioxide and water, the lactate-spilling process may accelerate - so much so that lactate levels in the blood may really begin to lift off. This point may be reached because not enough oxygen is getting into the cells to "handle" all the lactate (pyruvate) being produced, because there are not enough enzymes available to guide along the pyruvate-oxidation process, or because your muscle cells are somewhat lacking in "mitochondria" (mitochondria are the extremely tiny structures in which the key reactions of the Krebs cycle take place). It's very important to point out that this point may also be reached if your muscles and tissues are not very good at "clearing" large amounts of lactate from the blood once it appears there (more about this in a moment). Whatever the reason, the lactate-appearance rate in the blood may suddenly exceed the lactate-disappearance rate, and so your blood-lactate levels begin to climb somewhat precipitously. You have gone above your lactate threshold! Your lactate threshold (LT) velocity is simply the intensity (running, cycling, or swimming speed) above which lactate begins to accumulate in your blood.

OWEN ANDERSON

CHAPTER 5

LT IS THE BEST-POSSIBLE
PREDICTOR OF PERFORMANCE

As we mentioned in Chapter 4, your lactate threshold (LT) coincides with a very specific intensity of exercise (e. g., the intensity which causes lactate appearance to outstrip lactate disappearance). Bear in mind that the sudden lactate pile-up above LT is completely normal: Every single endurance athlete in the world has an LT; as workout difficulty increases, everyone eventually reaches an intensity at which lactate begins to burgeon in the blood. However, the speed at which LT occurs reveals a lot about how well you can function as an endurance athlete. If your LT is reached at a low running, cycling, or swimming speed, it often means that the "oxidative energy systems" in your muscles are not working very well. If they were performing at a high level, they would use oxygen to break lactate and pyruvate down to carbon dioxide and water, preventing lactate from pouring into the blood at such inchmeal paces.

As mentioned, a low LT might mean that you're not getting enough oxygen inside your muscle cells where it really matters. It might also mean that you don't have adequate concentrations of the enzymes necessary to oxidize lactate (pyruvate) at high rates, or that your mitochondria are in sorry shape. And since blood lactate depends not only on lactate formation but also on how well your tissues can utilize lactate once it appears, a low LT can also mean that your muscles, heart, and other tissues are not very good at *extracting* lactate from the blood.

In practical terms, you want to progressively move your LT to higher and higher running, cycling, or swimming speeds, because doing so will mean that your oxidative energy systems are improving and/or that your muscles are getting better at pulling lactate out of the blood and using it for energy. In effect, having a low LT is not bad in itself (as mentioned, the lactate won't hurt you), but it is a symptom that all is not well with your muscles' "machinery" for breaking down pyruvate, using oxygen, and clearing lactate from the blood.

There's also a very strong link between LT and how difficult your exercise *feels* to you. Any intensity above LT tends to feel pretty hard, while exerting yourself below LT is usually fairly comfortable. Thus, as LT rises, previously uncomfortable speeds suddenly begin to feel more sustainable, and you begin to complete your races at much faster paces.

In mathematical terms, there's a fairly tight connection between LT and competitive velocities. For example, if you're a runner, your 10-K race intensity is usually about 2.5 percent *above* your LT, while your-half-marathon speed can be no better than about 2.5 percent *below* LT. If you're really putting forth your best effort, and not just jogging through your races, those relationships are irrevocable, which means that without improving your LT, it would be absolutely impossible for you to run a half-marathon at your current best 10-K speed (after all, 10-K speed is above LT, and it's out of the question to run a half-marathon above LT intensity; you can't negotiate a race of that length any faster than 2.5 percent below your lactate threshold).

Generally, 5-K pace is about 2.5-percent faster than 10-K speed (and 5-percent quicker than LT), which brings up an interesting point. An absolute law of exercise is that the farther you stray above LT, the shorter will be the duration of your exertions; for example, 5-K pace, although just 2.5-percent hotter than 10-K striding, can be sustained for only 48 percent as long as 10-K pace. However, you shouldn't be depressed by the tight grip LT has on your performances: It's actually great news! LT is actually pretty easy to improve, and if you manage to heighten your LT by just 2.5 percent, your old 10-K pace will become your new half-marathon tempo, your old 5-K speed will become your new 10-K sizzling rate, and your new 5-K velocity will be 2.5 percent faster than your old 5-K PR! An upswing in LT means that you can hold your present race paces for longer periods of time - and boost your average race speeds. As your LT rises, so do your performances!

In fact, it's important to note that for most endurance athletes improving lactate threshold is *the* key to better performances. A variety of different scientific studies have shown that lactate threshold is the single best predictor of performance - better even than that vaunted physiological variable - VO$_2$max, *aka* maximal aerobic capacity ("Blood Lactate: Implications for Training and Sports Performance," *Sports Medicine*, vol. 3, pp. 10-25, 1986, and also "A Longitudinal Assessment of Anaerobic Threshold and Distance-Running Performance," *Medicine and Science in Sports and Exercise*, vol. 16(3), pp. 278-282, 1984).

People often wonder why LT is such a great fitness indicator and race predictor, but it's really not a big mystery. There are three key physiological variables which determine endurance performance - VO$_2$max, LT, and exercise economy (exercise economy is simply the efficiency with which an athlete moves at a particular speed; for example, if both cyclist A and cyclist B are racing each other at 20 miles per hour, but cyclist A requires 10 percent less energy (and oxygen) than B to hold that pace, then A is the more economical rider - and will usually win the race. Basically, athletes with enhanced economy are better able to conserve energy during competitions and also find fast paces to be less stressful, compared to athletes with poor economy.

You might think that VO2max would be the best predictor, since it's a reflection both of heart size and the muscles' ability to use oxygen to provide energy. If you've got a big pump (heart) and well-trained muscles, two things which are strongly correlated with good performances, your VO2max will indeed be pretty high. Indeed, elite male endurance athletes generally have VO2max readings above 75 ml/kg/min; elite females generally check in at 70 and above.

Still, VO2max is a coarse predictor of performance, because it doesn't tell you anything about economy. If a runner's VO2max is through the stratosphere but his/her economy is shoddy, performance may suffer mightily, and the runner might easily be beaten by another individual with a lower VO2max but more salubrious efficiency. For example, let's say that Jean and Ann are "duking it out" in a half-marathon, running at about the same rugged pace through the first eight miles of the race. Jean's VO2max is 78, while poor Ann checks in at "only" 70, so Jean should win, right? Well, hold on: As they fight it out, it "costs" Ann just 60 ml/kg/min of oxygen, which is 60/70 or 86 percent of her maximum. Meanwhile, Jean of the lofty VO2max is struggling; although she has kept pace so far, her efficiency is 20-percent worse than Ann's. Jean's actual cost is 72 ml/kg/min, or 92 percent of max, and so the pace *feels* much tougher to her than it does to Ann. In fact, Jean won't be able to continue much longer without slackening her pace, and Ann will go on to win, in spite of her lower VO2max. VO2max just doesn't contain enough information to be a great performance predictor. Economy isn't so good either, because it doesn't reveal anything about an athlete's VO2max, and it doesn't necessarily tell us very much about LT, either (please see "Ventilatory Threshold, Running Economy, and Distance Running Performance of Trained Athletes," *Research Quarterly for Exercise and Sports*, vol. 54, pp. 179-182, 1983). It's possible for an athlete to have pretty good economy but a mediocre LT - if he/she hasn't emphasized LT training very much.

LT, on the other hand, includes information about lactate dynamics *and* economy. Basically, it's impossible to have poor economy and a great LT simultaneously. That's because bad economy means that lots of energy must be used to maintain a particular pace, and high energy consumption usually means heavy-duty carbohydrate (glycogen and glucose) metabolism. Lots of glucose breakdown means big-time glycolysis and - you guessed it - very high lactate production. It's often difficult to have a great LT if lactate is spewing all over the place!

In contrast, great economy means minimal energy expenditure, a lower rate of carbohydrate metabolism, calmer rates of glycolysis, and reduced lactate production, which goes hand in hand with a nice LT. Thus, a runner with a fine LT is usually also one with a nifty economy, and that's why LT is such a foolproof performance predictor (it includes information about two of the three key predictors of endurance-performance success).

There's also great news (and certainly great news should be very welcome now that you've waded through all this physiology): Not only is LT the best predictor of performance, but it is also *very* responsive to training - much more responsive than VO2max in most experienced athletes. If you've been exercising regularly for several years, VO2max may not move upward at all over the course of a single training year, while LT might soar by up to 20 percent!

Remember Marc Rogers - our St.-Louis-Marathon winner (from Chapter 1)? You'll recall that Marc won the race not because of a big move in VO2max, which actually was static despite a very impressive training regime, but because of a huge lift-off in LT. Marc's "machinery" for oxidizing pyruvate and processing lactate improved dramatically, lifting his LT from 78 to 90 percent of VO2max, in less than four months of training. As a result, he was the one who took home the first-place trophy!

Why is LT so dynamic? "The skeletal muscles can adapt rather suddenly and strikingly to training, producing major gains in LT," says Marc, who is currently an exercise physiologist at the University of Maryland "In contrast, VO2max is a fairly stable cardiovascular variable in experienced endurance athletes. To understand that, bear in mind that VO2max is to a large degree dependent on the size of the left ventricle (the key heart chamber which pumps oxygenated blood out to the body), and the left ventricle just doesn't change very much in volume after you've been training for a number of years. That's why VO2max values may not rise at all - or may only increase by a couple of percent, even with a high volume and/or intensity of training. Meanwhile, LT can be expected to increase from 4 to 20 percent over the course of several months - given the appropriate training stimulus."

Scientific research strongly support's Marc's notion that VO2max can be a rather stubborn, static variable - while LT is extremely dynamic. When scientists at Georgia State University and the Emory University School of Medicine followed nine elite distance runners *over a two and one-half year period* during which the athletes prepared for the 1984 Summer Olympic Games in Los Angeles, they found that VO2max remained unchanged over the entire 30-month period, while LT advanced by an average of 6 percent. The LT upswing corresponded with either improved PRs or higher competitive rankings for the runners involved in the study ("Physiological Changes in Elite Male Distance Runners," *The Physician and Sportsmedicine*, vol. 14(1), pp. 152-171, 1986). Unfortunately, most endurance athletes don't realize how important LT training really is.

More Good News

As mentioned, another exciting aspect of LT improvement is that it seems to be much less limited by the aging process, compared with upswings in VO2max and economy ("Effects of Physical Training on Skeletal Muscle Metabolism and Ultrastructure in 70- to 75-Year-Old Men," *Acta Physiologica Scandinavica*, vol. 109, pp.

149-156, 1980, and also "Maintenance of the Adaptation of Skeletal Muscle Mitochondria to Exercise in Old Rats," *Medicine and Science in Sports and Exercise*, vol. 15, pp. 243-251, 1983). To put it another way, as you get older, your best *opportunity* for improving your performances may come from LT-type training.

That should not be a big shock. Remember that as you get older, maximal heart rate tends to decline by an average of one beat per year, and the strength and flexibility of the left ventricle, the heart's primary pump, also tend to diminish. These factors downgrade maximal cardiac output, a key component of VO2max. Meanwhile, those pesky little mitochondria which play a large role in enhancing LT (remember that they are the "stage" upon which pyruvate and lactate are broken down for energy via the Krebs cycle), and also the aerobic enzymes which give LT a kick-start, are not necessarily reduced by the aging process; in fact, they may increase almost as much in 60-year-old athletes as they would in competitors who are 30 years younger ("The Ageing Muscle," *Clinical Physiology*, vol. 3, pp. 209-218, 1983)!

The ability of older runners to make big advances in LT helps to explain a fascinating piece of research carried out several years ago by researchers at Washington University in St. Louis. In that investigation, eight masters athletes (average age 56) were compared with eight young runners (average age 25). Both groups ran the same number of miles per week (41) and also happened to have the same 10-K performance ability (average 10-K finishing time for young and old was around 41:30). As it turned out, VO_2max in the older competitors was almost *10-percent lower,* compared to the youngsters (again illustrating the poor predictive power of maximal aerobic capacity), and running economy was identical in the two groups. So why were the gray-haired harriers able to keep up with the rosy-cheeked saplings?

If you're guessing LT, you're right! Both the old and young runners reached LT at a speed of about 230 meters per minute (about seven minutes per mile), so it was no surprise that both groups ran their 10Ks at a pace of around 6:45 per mile (as we mentioned earlier, LT velocity and 10-K pace are predictably linked together). The higher VO_2max values of the younger runners were irrelevant for predicting performances (those lofty VO_2maxs should have foretold faster 10-K times for the young runners, but they didn't), because the LTs of the senior runners occurred at a higher percentage of VO_2max! In fact, average LT for the masters settled in at 85 percent of VO_2max, while LT for the striplings rested at only 79 percent of maximal aerobic capacity. As a result, the older runners were able to complete their 10Ks at about 88 to 90 percent of VO_2max, while the salad-days youngsters could only handle 81 percent (remember that runners can usually complete their 10-K races at an intensity which is just 2 to 3 percent above lactate-threshold intensity). You might be thinking that the older runners should have won the 10Ks (since their LTs were a higher percentage of VO_2max), but since they had lower VO_2maxs, 85 percent of their (lower) maximal aerobic capacities turned out to produce the same LT running speed as the younger runners' 79 percent of their (higher) VO2maxs. And since the two groups' LT *speeds* were the same, their performances in the 10K were also identical. For a detailed account of this fascinating research, please see "Lactate Threshold and Distance-Running Performance in Young and Older Endurance Athletes," *Journal of Applied Physiology*, vol. 58(4), pp. 1281-1284, 1985.

There's another important lesson here: If you're a masters athlete who is serious about maintaining or raising your level of performance, you need LT training (and advancement) even more than a younger athlete does. That's because after the age of 40 or so, VO2max begins a relentless decline which trims about 1/2 percent from your maximal aerobic capacity each year, even if you train extremely vigorously (if that seems like small potatoes, bear in mind that it adds up to a minimum of 5 percent in 10 years). The drop-off in VO2max is related to the fact that the heart becomes a stiffer, less potent pump as middle age progresses. Thus, the muscles are "showered" with less oxygen-rich blood during strenuous exercise, and VO2max edges downward. There's nothing you can do about this oxygen-utilization free-fall; your VO2max *is* going to diminish. However, you can compensate for the loss of aerobic capacity by continuing to improve your LT. Since LT is the most reliable predictor of performance, you can improve or maintain your performances as you get older by pushing LT steadily upward.

However, it really doesn't matter if you're young or old: You can and should work steadfastly on your lactate threshold! Giving your LT a hefty shove to a higher movement speed (e. g., to a higher percentage of your VO_2max) will allow you to keep pace with - and even beat- individuals who have higher maximal aerobic capacities than yours; it can also help you reach the PRs which you have always dreamed about. If you don't care about competing, heightening LT will allow you to train longer and more intensely than you ever have before, which will significantly upgrade your overall fitness and help you lose weight and improve your body composition.

CHAPTER 6

THE "HOW" AND "WHY"
OF LT TRAINING

So how do you actually cure a sickly LT - or take a pretty good LT and make it sensational? It's clear that there are two somewhat different ways to approach LT enhancement: First, you could work on increasing your muscle cells' "oxidative energy systems", e. g., their ability to take oxygen from the blood and use it to break down lactate (pyruvate) at very high rates. Of course, if lactate is broken down extremely rapidly, lots of energy will be produced, relatively modest amounts of lactate will spill into the blood, and the lucky athlete with such characteristics will be a highly fit, fast, strong competitor with a high LT. Enhancing the "oxidative energy systems" means improving the heart's capacity to deliver oxygen and the muscles' ability to use oxygen to break down lactate once the oxygen is delivered. This latter activity will necessitate both boosting the concentrations of aerobic enzymes inside muscle cells and augmenting the number of mitochondria within the muscle fibers.

However, the second approach is somewhat different: It involves augmenting the ability of the heart and muscles to "clear" lactate from the blood. You'll recall that lactate levels in the blood (and thus LT) are the result not only of the "appearance" of blood lactate (e. g., the rate at which it spills out of muscles into the bloodstream, which tends to reveal how well the oxidative energy systems are working) but also the "disappearance" of lactate (the rate at which muscles and the heart pull lactate out of blood plasma and break it down for energy). This disappearance rate - the ability of muscles to snare lactate from the blood - depends on a "carrier" protein called MCT1 (for monocarboxylate transporter 1). MCT1 attaches itself to muscle membranes and can help to transport (carry) lactate from the blood into the interior of muscle cells. The more MCT1 you have, the better you can "make lactate disappear" - and the higher should be your LT.

A key point: The workouts designed to optimally magnify MCT1 may be quite dissimilar from the "tried-and-true," traditional, LT-raising training sessions, and most endurance athletes fail to carry them out - and thus don't achieve their truly maximal LT. We'll describe how to actually carry out the MCT1 workouts in a moment.

What should you do to optimize your oxidative energy systems - and thereby boost your LT via the first mechanism described above? Runners and other endurance athletes have traditionally believed that prolonged, moderate exercise represents the ultimate LT therapy, and that's a fairly logical thought. After all, prolonged, medium-intensity exertions do tend to increase the muscles' ability to metabolize fat during exercise. If muscle fibers rely more heavily on fat and - therefore - less heavily on carbohydrate for fuel, less lactate will be produced (lactate is generated only from carbohydrate breakdown, not from fat degradation). Thus, at least in theory, less lactate "spilling" should take place, and LT should not be reached until a relatively high movement speed is attained.

But - hold on! There are many problems with this theory. As a practical point, moderate training speeds are dissimilar from actual racing speeds, and therefore it is difficult for the moderate-intensity trainer to develop good economy (efficiency of movement) at race velocities, since those higher speeds are not emphasized in training. To put it another way, moderately paced training is not very *specific* to racing, and the medium-intensity trainer seldom develops the great neuromuscular coordination patterns essential for excellent efficiency and first-rate racing.

In addition, even when an athlete develops a great fat-burning capacity, that capacity is seldom used in high-intensity racing situations. The problem is that fat becomes an increasingly minor source of energy at intensities above LT. Since most runners reach LT at about 10-mile (or 15-K) race speed, all shorter distances will be raced at intensities above LT. And of course this means that fat metabolism is pretty unimportant at distances of 10 miles or less, even in those athletes who have built up prodigious fat-burning furnaces. Thus, the huge training investment in long, slow miles rarely attenuates lactate production above LT (e. g., at race distances of 10 miles or less in runners), since fat can't "replace" carbohydrate at those intensities. In fact, high-volume, medium-intensity training may actually aggrandize lactate appearance above LT, because the muscles of athletes who train that way are relatively unschooled at clearing and processing lactate. It certainly does not seem to be the way to maximize your ability to handle lactate.

Not surprisingly, scientific research reveals that fairly intense training is the best booster of LT. But before we get into this research, we should mention that another popular method for raising LT - doing a lot of training at an intensity which produces a blood-lactate level of 4 mmol/liter - is also questionable. 4-mmol training became popular, especially among swimming coaches, about two decades ago when it became apparent that a reading of 4 mmol/liter was at - or slightly above - lactate threshold in a fair number of endurance athletes. The idea was simply that by training "at the limit of the lactate system" (e. g., at the "lactate threshold" of 4 mmol/liter), as it was often expressed, one could increase the chances of strengthening the "system" and boosting LT.

This is very tenuous thinking, however. For one

thing, a reading of 4 mmol/liter is not really at the limit of the lactate-producing system; in fact, it is often the point at which lactate production really begins to take off. It's not even the limit of the "lactate-containment" system, if you prefer to think of the threshold in that way, because lactate clearance is actually much more dramatic at higher exercise intensities and blood-lactate readings. It's just that lactate production is so lofty at the higher intensities that the expansive clearance rate can't quite keep pace, and so blood-lactate readings tend to rise.

Another problem with 4 mmol-training is that many athletes can exercise comfortably and without apparent fatigue or stress even though their blood-lactate levels may be at 6 or even 7 mmol/liter, well above the 4-mmol mark. These stable, comfortable lactate readings (of 6 to 7 mmol/liter) indicate that these athletes have not yet reached their LT, even though they are well above the 4-mmol "standard." Attempting to boost LT by training at the intensity which coincides with 4-mmol/liter lactate concentrations would be foolhardy for such athletes, since they would be actually be training *below* LT - and thus creating too weak a stimulus to propel LT upward.

That being said, we should note that 4-mmol training can improve LT in *some* athletes - specifically in those who reach LT at a lower lactate level, but it is by no means the best way to produce a really impressive LT, even for those people whose LT is sub-4 mmol/liter.

As mentioned, scientific research strongly supports the idea that intense work (at and especially above LT) is best for hoisting LT. In a study carried out at the University of North Carolina at Greensboro, runners who suddenly raised their average training intensity by completing two fartlek sessions and one interval workout per week boosted LT significantly in just eight short weeks and shaved over a minute from average 10-K time. The fartlek work involved two- to five-minute bursts at 10-K pace, which is about 2 to 3 percent faster than LT speed; the intervals were completed at about 5-K speed, which is around 6 percent quicker than LT velocity ("Increased Training Intensity Effects on Plasma Lactate, Ventilatory Threshold, and Endurance," *Medicine and Science in Sports and Exercise*, vol. 21(5), pp. 563-568, 1989).

The idea that intense workouts are best for boosting LT was even more strongly reinforced in research carried out at York University by Stephen Keith and Ira Jacobs ("Adaptations to Training at the Individual Anaerobic Threshold," *Medicine and Science in Sports and Exercise*, vol. 23(4), Supplement, #197, 1991). In the York investigations, one group of athletes trained exactly *at* their current LT, a very popular form of LT training, for 30 minutes per workout. A second group of exercisers divided their 30-minute workouts into four intervals, each of which lasted for seven and one-half minutes. Two of the intervals were completed at an intensity *above* LT, while the other two were carried out below LT. Each group of athletes worked out four times per week for a total of eight weeks.

In the second group, the "below-LT" exertions (which were used for two of the four 7.5-minute intervals per workout) corresponded with an intensity of about 60 to 73 percent of VO2max, a very moderate level of effort which is used by many endurance athletes during their long, slow workouts and easy, shorter training sessions - and which is unlikely to have much impact on LT. The "above-LT" intensity (also used for two 7.5-minute intervals per workout) was set at about 30 percent of the difference between lactate threshold and actual VO2max. 30 percent of the LT-VO2max difference would actually represent an intensity of up to 87 percent of VO2max, or about 88 to 93 percent of maximal heart rate. In terms of actual running velocity, it would correspond to a running speed which is almost exactly the same as 10-K pace (or perhaps a few seconds per mile slower). In contrast, actual LT intensity is more like 15-K to 10-mile race pace.

Which strategy was better for boosting LT - working *at* LT intensity or putting in the time above it? After eight weeks of workouts, both sets of athletes achieved similar increases in VO2max and LT. The actual gains in LT were absolutely tremendous, averaging 14 percent in both groups!! Advances in aerobic enzymes were also rather impressive - and nearly identical in the two groups. In an endurance test in which group members exercised for as long as possible at an intensity which corresponded to their pre-training LT, the above-LT trainees seemed to hold an edge, sustaining their exercise for a total of 71 minutes, while the at-LT subjects could last for only 64 minutes. However, this difference was not statistically significant.

At first glance, these results seem to suggest that there's not much advantage to be gained by surging through highly demanding, above-LT workouts, but wait! If you've been following along, you probably noticed that the above-LT athletes really logged only 60 minutes of *quality* work per week (4 X 15 minutes per workout; we won't count their easy, below-LT exertions), while the at-LT subjects put in 120 weekly minutes of quality exertion (4 X 30 minutes). To put it another way, the above-LT athletes achieved the same gains in LT and VO2max as the at-LT folks (and perhaps enjoyed a slight advantage in endurance) - with only half the total quality training time! It's reasonable to assume that had the above-LT athletes stepped up their volume of above-LT work a little bit, they would have outdistanced the mundane at-LT trainees.

What Happens Above LT?

Why does roaming above LT during training seem to be so effective at lifting lactate threshold? For one thing, as illustrated by the York University research, such roaming has a dramatic impact on the aerobic enzymes required to break down lactate and pyruvate (remember that 60 weekly minutes above LT were as good as 120 minutes at LT, in terms of increasing muscle-cell enzymes). Investigations carried out with laboratory animals demonstrate another reason why above-LT exertions work so well. In research carried out at the University of Missouri, several groups of rats hustled along on laboratory treadmills at a variety of different paces, which ranged from 15 to 37 meters per minute (43 to 100 minutes per mile). The faster (by rat standards) velocities (e. g., those speeds of approximately 30 meters per minute and above) produced a flood-tide of lactate in the rodents' bloodstreams, as expected, but the Missouri researchers also noticed something very interesting: High lactate levels were linked with glycogen depletion of the rats' "fast-twitch" muscle fibers, not their "slow-twitch" cells. In other words, fast-twitch fibers were primarily responsible for the huge upswing in blood lactate ("New Workout Helps Lift Your Lactate Threshold toward VO2max," *Running Research News*, vol. 7(4), pp. 1, 4-5, 1991).

Of course, fast-twitch fibers aren't heavily utilized during moderately paced exertions but play a larger and larger role as movement speeds increase beyond LT pace. Compared to their slow-twitch brethren, these fast-twitch guys are ordinarily somewhat low on mitochondria and aerobic enzymes, so it makes sense that they would begin belching out lactate as they are called into play. If they are very, very poor at oxidizing pyruvate, massive amounts of lactic acid will be produced, and LT will be reached at a very mediocre pace. As they get better at breaking down pyruvate, less lactate will be produced and LT speed will of course increase, but there's only one way to stimulate the fast-twitchers to get better: It's to *use* them during training, specifically at fairly sustained, fast paces. To put it another way, fast-twitch muscle cells can be the "culprits" behind a low LT, and the only way to upgrade their oxygen-processing machinery is to hammer away at them during training. You'll get more "bang from your buck" with faster-paced training, compared to slower efforts, because it forces the fast-twitchers to do their "homework".

What if your muscle fibers are primarily slow-twitch? Does the same intensity argument still apply? Again, bear in mind that the key problem associated with a low LT is an inability of muscle cells to oxidize pyruvate and lactate at high rates. The only way to teach them to handle pyruvate and lactate quickly is to expose them to higher concentrations of those common compounds, and that means fast-paced training, regardless of whether the cells are slow or fast twitchers. Remember that faster training revs up glycolysis, which can literally flood muscle cells with pyruvate and lactate.

The advantages of higher-intensity training were also illustrated by research completed at the State University of New York at Syracuse. In this study, which was carried out over an eight-week period, the concentration of a mitochondrial enzyme called cytochrome c increased by about *1 percent per minute* of daily LT training, as long as training intensity was set at 85 to 100 percent of VO_2max, or approximately 92 to 100 percent of maximal heart rate. This means that by carrying out 10 minutes of daily training within this intensity zone, subjects boosted cytochrome c by 10 percent after eight weeks; with 27 minutes of daily training within the high-intensity zone, cytochrome c advanced by 27 percent in eight weeks. In contrast, working at a lower intensity of only 70 to 75 percent of VO2max increased cytochrome c by only 2/3 percent per minute of daily training. Since cytochrome c is a critically important oxidative enzyme found within the mitochondria, upswings in cytochrome c should be fairly well correlated with improvements in LT.

In this SUNY-Syracuse study, if one looked at fast-twitch muscle fibers only, the gains associated with faster training were even more impressive: 10 minutes of daily training at 100 percent VO2max roughly *tripled* cytochrome c concentrations within fast-twitch cells, while running 27 minutes per day at 85 percent VO2max expanded cytochrome c by just 80 percent, and *90* daily minutes at 70 percent VO2max burgeoned cytochrome c by just 74 percent ("Influence of Exercise Intensity and Duration on Biochemical Adaptations in Skeletal Muscle," *Journal of Applied Physiology,* vol. 53(4), pp. 844-850, 1982).

A Range of Optimal Intensities

Overall, the scientific research suggests that - for runners - the range of intensities from about 5-K pace down to about 10-mile race pace is great for improving LT, with the faster paces within this zone being "better" for raising LT when the improvement is plotted as a gain per minute of training (we'll discuss the optimal intensities for cyclists and swimmers a bit later in the book). However, in fairness we should mention that a potential advantage of the "slower" paces (e. g., those close to 10-mile race speed) within this zone is that they can often be used for many more minutes of weekly training, compared to the faster paces, possibly counteracting their "per minute disadvantage" (for example, it is much easier to complete 45 minutes of training at one's 10-mile race pace during a week of training than it is to charge through a total of 45 minutes of work intervals at 5-K pace, and the risk of overtraining and injury is probably also lower with a more moderate speed).

In addition, the "slower" paces within the LT zone may be used to create longer work intervals during interval training and may also be sustained for 25 to 35 minutes of *continuous* running. Both the long work intervals (of 2000 to 3000 meters) and the sustained running (25 to 35 minutes) help runners develop the ability to *maintain* quality velocities for longer periods of time, as they must do during races. In contrast, shorter intervals may feature a higher, more LT-productive intensity but don't simulate race situations as well (after all, few races permit recovery intervals!).

Supporting the idea that the moderate end of the LT zone can be great for spurring performance, research carried out at Charles University in Prague, Czechoslovakia determined that runners improved their LTs and performances most dramatically when they augmented the amount of weekly running carried out at velocities which fell between 10-K and 10-mile race speeds (10-K velocity is about 2 to 3 percent above LT pace, while 10-mile velocity is very close to actual LT speed, as mentioned). In this Czech research, a group of seven experienced runners downgraded the amount of aerobic training they carried out from 80 to 72 percent of all miles over a four-month period (aerobic workouts were defined as those conducted at a pace slower than 10-mile race speed). Meanwhile, the quantity of LT training (defined as runs of five miles or less at a pace somewhere between 10-K and 10-mile race speeds) advanced substantially from 6 to 16 percent of all miles (the remaining, basically unchanging volume of 12 to 14 percent was always reserved for short, speedy intervals on the track at faster than 10-K pace). As a result of the increase in LT-type training, LT velocity improved by a full 10 percent in four months, and 10-K race times sharpened by almost a half-minute - from 28:45 to 28:20 ("Ventilatory Threshold and Mechanical Efficiency in Endurance Runners," *European Journal of Applied Physiology*, vol. 58, pp. 693-698, 1989).

It *is* important to note that the more temperate end of the LT training zone (e. g., paces which are closer to 10-mile than to 5-K race velocity) seems to work best when these "cooler" paces are sustained in a continuous manner for periods of 20 minutes or more. An example of this is the classic study carried out at the famed Karolinska Institute in Stockholm, Sweden many years ago. In this research, Swedish runners added just one thing to their usual training - a weekly 20-minute run completed at a pace which was about 10 to 12 seconds *slower* per mile than 10-K race speeds, which happens to be just about 10-mile race speed, or the "bottom end" of the LT zone. After a total of 14 weeks, the Swedes'

LTs improved by 4 percent, and 10-K times were trimmed by over a minute ("Changes in Onset of Blood Lactate Accumulation (OBLA) and Muscle Enzymes after Training at OBLA," *European Journal of Applied Physiology*, vol. 49, pp. 45-57, 1982).

In addition to being a nice duration for a moderately long, LT-boosting effort, 20 minutes may also be very close to the threshold for the amount of weekly LT-type work needed to heighten LT significantly. Research at the University of Ulm in Germany has determined that investing 20 to 25 minutes or more per week in LT training can lead to large LT lift-offs, while completing less than that quantity of weekly LT work is linked with mediocre thresholds ("German Runners Find Right Dose of Threshold Running," *Running Research News*, vol. 8(4), pp. 1-3, 1992).

CHAPTER 7

THE MYSTERIOUS MCT1

So far, we've pointed out that the optimal intensity zone for LT improvement seems to be about 85 to 100 percent VO2max (for runners, this roughly means between 10-mile and 5-K race speeds). Training within this zone produces a variety of adaptations which lessen lactate production, including better oxygen delivery to muscles, increased numbers of mitochondria, and heightened levels of mitochondrial enzymes. We'll show you how to construct workouts within this optimal zone in Chapter 10.

However, you'll recall that another key part of the LT-lifting story involves enhancing lactate clearance (aka lactate disappearance). The basic idea behind this is simply that even after you've minimized lactate production and lifted your LT, you're still going to get into situations (during races and tough workouts) in which you're going to be above LT, and therefore producing a fair amount of lactate. If you can learn to "clear" this lactate, you'll have more fuel available to exercise at a high intensity. Furthermore, a great lactate-clearance capacity "postpones" LT, allowing it to coincide with a faster speed of movement.

For many years, exercise scientists weren't certain that it would actually be possible to improve the ability of muscles to seize especially large quantities of lactate and then break the lactate down for fuel. However, in 1993 a study carried out by lactate expert Arend Bonen and his research group at the University of Waterloo in Ontario, Canada showed that muscles could indeed learn to "clear" lactate at advanced rates, provided the training stimulus was appropriate ("Endurance Training Increases Skeletal Muscle Lactate Transport," *Acta Physiologica Scandinavica*, vol. 147(3), pp. 323-327, 1993). At that time, no one knew *how* the muscles were actually transporting more lactate, however.

But Bonen and his research crew kept at it, and in 1996 they discovered a unique muscle-cell protein called MCT1 (for monocarboxylate transporter 1). Bonen and his colleagues were able to show that MCT1 is indeed a "lactate transporter"; it can actually move lactate into muscle cells, where of course the lactate can be broken down to provide energy for high-intensity exercise ("Role of the Lactate Transporter (MCT1) in Skeletal Muscles," *American Journal of Physiology*, vol. 271 *(Endocrinology and Metabolism 34)*, pp. E143-150, 1996).

Bonen has published more work since then, and

his research makes for extremely fascinating reading. His key findings to date can be summarized in this way:

(1) You *can not* increase lactate uptake by muscle cells unless you first increase concentrations of MCT1. There's no getting around it!

(2) Both the muscles and the heart can increase their levels of MCT1 rather dramatically (as it turns out, the heart is a big "burner" of lactate).

(3) MCT1 levels can respond fairly quickly to training, increasing by as much as 18 percent in seven days. However, the potential improvements in MCT1 are much greater when longer periods of training are utilized.

What intensity of exercise is best for spiking MCT1 production? Research in this area is still in its infancy, but so far it suggests that very high intensities may be superior. In Bonen's most recent study, laboratory rats were divided into two different groups, both of which trained for three weeks. One group exercised moderately - at a pace of only 21 meters per minute with a treadmill grade of 8 percent. The second collection of rats trained intensely - at a relatively sizzling speed of 31 meters per minute with the treadmill jacked up to 15 percent ("Training Intensity-Dependent and Tissue-Specific Increases in Lactate Uptake and MCT-1 in Heart and Muscle," *Journal of Applied Physiology*, vol. 84(3), pp. 987-994, 1998).

After three weeks, the moderately trained rodents failed to raise their muscular concentrations of MCT1 at all! Not surprisingly, lactate uptake was also no better than before. In contrast, the intensely trained rats augmented MCT1 levels in key muscles by 70 to 94 percent and boosted lactate uptake by around 80 percent.

The more intense training also benefited the heart to a greater extent. After three weeks of moderate training, heart MCT1 was up by 36 percent, and heart lactate uptake increased by 72 percent. In contrast, after three weeks of intense training, heart MCT1 advanced by 44 percent, and heart lactate uptake ballooned by 173 percent!

This early research strongly supports the notion that highly intense training is best for boosting MCT1 and lactate uptake, and it seems quite logical that this would be the case. The most potent stimulus for increasing MCT1 levels may in fact be high blood- and muscle-lactate levels (just as the best stimulus for improving VO_2max is to use oxygen at very high rates), You can't have high lactate levels unless you exercise very intensely.

High-intensity workouts which involve fairly heavy lactate outputs should also improve the "buffering capacity" of muscles, e. g., their ability to cope with the upward zooms in acidity associated with very intense exercise. These acid "rushes" are associated with kicks to the finish line at the ends of races, mid-race surges to lose troublesome opponents, and lung-searing hill climbs during race efforts and hill workouts. They can also occur when you start your races or workouts too quickly; without good buffering capacity, you may not recover enough to finish your competition or training session in a quality way.

Research carried out at Iowa State University indicates that athletes can improve their lactate-clearance and muscle-buffering capacities by conducting workouts which essentially consist of 45- to 120-second intervals carried out *at close to maximal intensity*, with two- to four-minute recoveries between intervals ("Lactic Acid Tolerance Training: Floods of Lactic Acid Aren't Necessarily Bad - If You Can Endure Them, *Running Research News*, vol. 8(6), pp. 1-4, 1992). Of course, the purpose of the short blasts of exertion is to produce lots of lactate, while the rationale for the relatively long recoveries is to coax the muscle cells into increasing their ability to metabolize the lactate produced during the work intervals - as well as provide enough "down" time so that the next work interval can be conducted at a very hard intensity which "spills out" another dense batch of lactate. Such sessions should significantly heighten MCT1 concentrations. More information about these workouts, as well as instructions for including the MCT1 sessions in your overall LT training, are included in Chapter 10.

OWEN ANDERSON

CHAPTER 8

STRENGTH TRAINING
FOR LT IMPROVEMENT

When we think about creating optimal LT-boosting workouts, we usually imagine running, cycling, or swimming at certain speeds. However, research has indicated that strength training (in the form of "circuits" of various exercises) can also have a positive impact on LT. In research carried out at the University of Maryland, 10 individuals participated in a 12-week strength-training program, while a control group of eight subjects avoided strengthening activities. The strength trainees carried out their fortifying workouts three times a week, and their circuits of 10 different exercises were completed three times per workout, adding up to a total of nine circuits per week. The 10 exertions in each circuit included hip flexions, knee extensions, knee flexions, leg presses, parallel squats, bent-knee sit-ups, bench presses, push-ups, lat pull-downs, and arm curls. 15 to 20 reps of each exercise were completed per circuit (e. g., there were 45 to

60 reps of each exercise per workout).

After 12 weeks, there was no change at all in VO2max, but the resistance exercisers did improve quadriceps and hamstring strength dramatically and bolstered endurance time during an intense exercise test by about 33 percent (from 26 to 35 minutes). Most impressively, LT advanced by a full 12 percent ("Effects of Strength Training on Lactate Threshold and Endurance Performance," *Medicine and Science in Sports and Exercise*, vol. 23(6), pp. 739-743, 1991).

Why did the circuits hoist LT upward? In an interview with the author of *Lactate Lift-Off*, the key researcher involved in the study, Ben Hurley, Ph. D., theorized that "resistance training improved the power of individual muscle cells, so not as many powerful "fast-twitch" fibers needed to be recruited during exercise." Since fast-twitch cells are notorious for producing lots of lactate, their reduced activation should lead to lower lactate outputs during exertion and thus a potentially higher lactate threshold.

However, there's also another possibility: As muscular strength increases, better whole-body stability can be achieved during exercise (there is less unnecessary motion during activity because of the stabilizing effect of stronger muscles). As whole-body stableness improves, there is a reduced need to "waste" energy compensating for unnecessary motions (e. g., to expend energy to bring the body back into proper position for optimal movement). Thus, a greater percentage of muscular force production can be channeled into forward propulsion, rather than the correction of "sloppiness". This should heighten one's movement speed at all fractions of VO2max, including LT, and thus raise LT velocity.

However, it's important to note that the strength routines which are most likely to hike LT are the ones which upgrade whole-body strength, such as push-ups and feet-elevated push-ups, body-weight squats, squat thrusts with jumps (burpees), squat and dumbbell presses, bench dips, "core exercises," and lunges, as well as exertions which closely mimic the movements involved in your sport (if you're a runner, these exercises would include one-leg squats, high-bench step-ups, and one-leg hops in place). The reasoning for this is simple: If you don't strengthen your whole body, some portion of your anatomy may remain weak - and energy-wasteful during exercise. In addition, if you don't utilize at least a few exercises which tightly parallel the neuromuscular demands of your sport, you'll never develop optimal coordination and stability during the precise movements associated with your preferred activity. Routines which isolate muscles, which are non-weight bearing, or which are poorly related to the biomechanics of your sport (e. g., single-joint movements on weight machines) are probably much less likely to benefit LT.

It's also important to note that the circuits of whole-body exercises designed to hike LT should also include some actual running (or cycling or swimming) intervals. The reason for this, of course, is that the intervals will force the muscle fibers which are most critical to your success in your goal activity (running, cycling, or swimming) to "clear" lactate and break it down for energy (some of this lactate will be generated by the strengthening exercises which are also part of the circuits). The intervals are also great for your mental toughness and confidence; by completing the intervals even when you are dog-tired from the strengthening exercises, you soon learn that you can run at goal pace even when your muscles are gripped by almost-paralyzing fatigue. Finally, the intervals can be used to spike the overall intensity of the workout (remember that higher intensity is the most potent producer of lofty LTs).

The LT-Enhancing Circuit

Here is just one example of an LT-boosting circuit workout:

Please warm up with 15 minutes of moderate, continuous exercise, and then perform the following activities in the order indicated. Move quickly from exercise to exercise, but don't perform the exercises themselves overly quickly (don't sacrifice good form just to get them done in a hurry). The idea is to do each exercise methodically and efficiently - and then almost immediately start on the next exertion.

(1) Run 400 meters at your 5-K race pace (or cycle or swim for one to two minutes at an intensity which would rate a 9 or 9.5 on an effort scale of 1 to 10, with 1 being the easiest-possible exercise and 10

being maximal exertion).

       (2) Do 4 chin-ups.

       (3) Complete 30 ab crunches.

       (4) Perform 12 push-ups.

       (5) Complete 15 squat thrusts with jumps (burpees).

       (6) Perform 30 body-weight squats (fast).

       (7) Run 400 meters at 5-K pace (or cycle or swim, as indicated).

       (8) Do 10 squat and dumbbell presses (w. 10-pound dumbbells).

       (9) Perform 8 feet-elevated push-ups.

       (10) Complete 30 low-back extensions.

       (11) Perform 15 bench dips.

       (12) Complete 15 lunges with each leg.

       (13) Run 400 meters at 5-K pace (or cycle or swim).

       (14) Repeat steps 2-13 one more time (for two circuits in all), and then cool down with 10 to 15 minutes of easy activity.

       This circuit workout seems remarkably easy on paper, but it can be challenging to carry out! Over time, the session can be progressively stiffened by increasing the number of reps of the various exercises, lengthening the running, cycling, or swimming intervals, and increasing the total number of circuits from two to three - and then four. You can carry out the circuits a couple of times a week during an early phase of your training cycle to get your LT started upward, and you can also "blend" the circuits with other forms of LT training during those periods when you are really emphasizing LT development (please see the chapter on LT workouts for full details). Overall, the circuits should have a very positive impact on your running fitness, overall strength, and especially LT!

Core Strengthening
to Improve LT

It's also reasonable to expect that improving the strength of your "core" muscles - the muscles attached to your pelvic girdle and lower spine - should help upgrade your LT, too. To understand the importance of your core muscles, which include your "abs" and low-back muscles, think of your body as a chain made up of just three links. The two end links represent your legs, while the middle link consists of your pelvic girdle and trunk. As you run, you transfer force from one leg to the other, and the only possible path of force transference is through the middle link (your core). If your middle link is weak, it's like putting a wet, floppy noodle in between two powerful steel cables, and it will be impossible for you to transfer force efficiently from one leg to the other.

In addition, all of the key upper-leg muscles used in running are attached to the core - the pelvic girdle or spine. If that core is not held in stable, proper position by the core muscles, the leg muscles simply do not have a strong "anchor point" from which they can contract powerfully.

When you run, your butt muscles and hamstrings, all of which are attached to your pelvic girdle, drive your leg backward and your body forward at the end of the "stance" phase of the gait cycle (just before toe-off). As this happens, the core muscles in your abdominal area must prevent your torso from flopping backward (to picture this, remember that inertia tries to keep your upper body from moving forward as your leg creates thrust). When you land on your opposite foot, the core muscles in your lower back must decelerate your upper body to keep it from pitching forward.

In addition to thwarting this energy-squandering, backward-and-forward floppiness, your core muscles keep your upper body from waggling from side to side as you gambol along (the basic problem is that each time your right foot hits the ground, there's a tendency for your upper body to lurch to the left, and vice-versa). Your core muscles also control the key rotational movements involved in running. Although you may think of running as a straight-ahead activity, with movement occurring in only one plane, the truth is that when your left leg moves forward, your left hip rotates in a clockwise manner while your right shoulder rotates in a counter-clockwise fashion. When your right leg moves ahead, your right hip rotates counter-clockwise and your left shoulder moves clockwise. These rotational movements are coordinated and stabilized by your core muscles to keep your upper body from behaving like an out-of-control washtub, which would waste tremendous amounts of energy (for example, if your trunk twisted too far in one direction, excessive energy would be required to rotate it back to a neutral, straight-ahead position with each stride).

How does all of this relate to LT? As mentioned, if your upper body is not stable, extra energy must be expended to stabilize it. If your leg muscles do not have a strong anchor point against which they can produce propulsive force, extra energy will be needed to drive your body forward. Much of this extra energy will come from the breakdown of carbohydrate, so glycolysis will proceed more intensely, and surplus lactate will be more likely to appear in your muscles and blood. If you increase your intensity of exercise, additional energy will be required to stabilize your body, and even more lactate will appear. The unfortunate consequence is that you will reach LT at a very modest movement speed, compared to the stable, well-coordinated athlete who is expending less energy to maintain good body control. The athlete with great core strength can attain higher speeds without going over threshold.

So how do you advance core strength? One of the very best core exercises is as follows:

(A) Lie down on the ground or floor and stretch out in a prone position (with face and belly downward). Then, lift up your body so that full body weight is supported only by your forearms and toes. In this position, your elbows are on the ground and should be almost directly below your shoulders. Your forearms and hands are resting on the ground, pointed straight ahead (parallel to the line made by your body). Your toes (and feet) are about shoulder-width apart, and your toes are the only part of your lower body which are in contact the ground. Your whole body is supported only by your forearms and toes.

(B) Then, "tuck" your pelvis. This basically means rotating your pelvic girdle by pushing the lower part of your pelvic area toward the ground while the upper part of the pelvis rotates away from the ground. Your hip area doesn't actually come any closer to the ground (your whole body should be in a fairly straight line from your toes up to your shoulders). When you "tuck", you are just rotating your pelvis, not moving it up or down. If you were standing, you would be directing the lower part of your pelvis forward and pulling the top part of your pelvic girdle backward. If you think of your pelvic girdle as a bowl of milk, you would be tipping that bowl backward, so that milk could pour out of the back side of the bowl. As strange as this may seem, this tucking action is critically important if you want to gain the full benefit of the exercise.

(C) Hold this basic position (body supported only on forearms and toes, pelvis tucked) for 15 seconds, and then lift your right arm off the ground, straighten it, and point it straight ahead, holding it in the air for 10 seconds (at this point, your body is supported only by your left forearm and the toes of your two feet). After 10 seconds, return to the starting position.

(D) Then, lift your left arm off the ground and point it straight ahead, holding it in the air for 10 seconds (your body is supported only by your toes and right forearm). Return to the starting position.

(E) Now lift your right leg off the ground and hold it there (roughly parallel with the ground) for 10 seconds (your body will now be supported by your two forearms and the toes on your left foot). Return to the starting position.

(F) Lift your left leg in the air and hold it parallel with the ground for 10 seconds, and then return to the starting position.

(G) *Here's a move you'll always remember:* From the basic starting position, lift your right arm and left leg in the air *simultaneously* (your body will now be supported only by your right toes and left forearm). Hold them up for 10 seconds, and then return to the starting position.

F. Then, lift your left arm and right leg *simultaneously,* and hold them in the air for 10 seconds. Return to the starting position.

Take a one-minute break, and then return to the basic starting position and repeat steps A-F one more time. Sorry!

Once you've completed the second series, stay in the basic position, supported on forearms and toes only, and hold this basic position for two full minutes! Maintain an absolutely straight body posture for the entire two-minute period.

You're almost done! But before stopping the core exercise, flip over onto your back for a moment. This time, lift your body off the ground by supporting full body weight with only the *heels* of your feet and your forearms (as a variation on this, you can also try supporting your upper body with your hands). Once again, try to keep your body in a fairly linear position, and remember to tuck your pelvis! Follow the same movement pattern outlined above (lifting first your left arm, and then your right arm, left leg, and right leg in succession). Then, you can try lifting your left arm and right leg together, and then your right arm and left leg together. It's also fun to do more than just lift your appendages. For example, you can move an arm back and forth in a running-like motion or bring a knee toward your chest or swing your leg from side to side to increase the "loading" and stress on your core muscles.

Finally, flip over onto your right side and support full body weight with only your right forearm and the outside of your right foot. The direction of your forearm should be roughly perpendicular to the line of your body. Initially, your left leg is merely lying on top of your right leg, but the idea is to lift the left leg up in the air for about 20 seconds. Once you've done this, return the left leg to the basic position, rest for a moment, and repeat. Then, shift over to your left side and repeat this pattern (full body weight supported only by left forearm and outside of left foot), lifting your right leg in the air for about 20 seconds at a time. You can increase the difficulty of this portion of the core exercise by moving the air-borne legs to the front and back as your body remains in a stable position.

How often should you carry out this core routine? Drop down into a prone position at parties and impress your friends and relatives with your core strength. Carry out the core exertions in your office in-between humdrum meetings. When conversation bottoms out at the family dinner table, hit the floor and amaze your spouse and children with your unusual new ability. This routine can be carried out nearly everyday as a healthy break from your various duties, and it's a terrific way to strengthen your core. If you complete the core exertions faithfully, you'll soon be much stronger in the middle of your body, and your LT should be more robust, too.

Special Exercises to Improve LT

If you're a runner, performance of three special exercises which mimic the neuromuscular patterns associated with running should also aid LT. By developing greater strength during running-specific motions, you will have increased stability while running and therefore lower energy expenditure and lactate production. However, there's also a second benefit: When you strengthen your leg and hip muscles in a manner specific to running, you are basically strengthening the individual muscle cells which make up those key muscles. Once individual cells are stronger, *fewer* cells are required to sustain a specific running pace; thus, energy consumption and total lactate production are lower while running, and LT consequently shifts to a higher running speed.

The three key exercises - **one-leg squats, high-bench step-ups, and one-leg hops in place** - should be performed only when you are well rested. Always remember that specific strength training aims for positive adaptations of the nervous system as well as the muscles. Completing the exercises when you are overly fatigued leads to poor neuromuscular coordination - and movements which are slower than desirable.

That means that the trio of specific exercises should usually be completed before a running workout, not after, and in fact the best-possible time is immediately *prior* to an interval, economy, or lactate-threshold session, not before a slower workout. While that may sound paradoxical (some would fear that strength training would slow down a subsequent training session), the truth is that positioning the exercises right before your high-intensity exertion will help you run *faster*. In fact, at least five different scientific studies have shown that a high-intensity strength session activates the nervous system, increases the "firing rate" of nerve cells which control muscles, and improves the overall "recruitment" of muscle fibers during a workout (please see Paavo Komi's article "The Stretch-Shortening Cycle and Human Power Output," in L. Jones, N. McCartney, and A. McComas, eds., *Human Muscle Power*, pp. 27-42, Human Kinetics, Champaign, Illinois).

Please perform the one-leg hops in place only on an aerobics floor, wooden gym floor, grass, a rubberized track, or any resilient surface which offers some "give." Hopping repeatedly on concrete or asphalt may increase the risk of overuse injuries to the lower leg and shin.

Here's how to perform the three key exercises:

(1) THE HIGH-BENCH STEP-UP: This exercise strongly develops the hamstrings, with complimentary development of the gluteals (the "butt" muscles) and the quadriceps. Simply begin from a standing position on top of a high bench (approximately knee height), with your body weight on your left foot and your weight shifted toward the left heel. The right foot should be free and held slightly behind the body. Lower your body in a controlled manner until the toes of the right foot touch the ground, but maintain all of your weight on the left foot. Return to the starting position by driving downward with the left heel and straightening the left leg. Repeat for about 10 repetitions, and then switch over to the right leg. Maintain absolutely upright posture with the trunk throughout the entire movement, with your hands held at your sides (with or without dumbbells).

(2) ONE-LEG SQUAT: This exercise strongly develops the quadriceps and gluteals, with a complimentary boost to the hamstrings. To complete one-leg squats in the correct way, stand with your left foot forward and the right foot back, with the feet about one shin-length apart from front to back (your feet should be hip-width apart from side to side). Place the toes of the right foot on a block or step which is six to eight inches high. As in the step-up exercise, most of the weight should be directed through the heel of the left foot. Bend the left leg and lower the body until the left knee reaches an angle of 90 degrees between the thigh and lower leg. Return to the starting position, maintaining upright posture with the trunk and holding your hands at your sides. Complete about 10 repetitions with the left leg before switching to the right leg.

(3) ONE-LEG HOPS IN PLACE: This exercise builds strength and coordination in the entire lower extremity, including the foot, ankle, shin, calf, thigh, and hip. The resilient, bouncy nature of the exercise makes it the most specific of the three - extremely close to the actual movements involved in running. Simply start from the same position you used for the one-leg squat, with the toes of the right foot supported by a six- to eight-inch block. Hop rapidly on the left foot at a cadence of 2.5 to 3 hops per second (25 to 30 foot contacts per 10 seconds) for the prescribed time period for about 20 seconds. The left knee should rise about four to six inches, while the right leg and foot should remain completely stationary. The left foot should strike the ground in the area of the mid-foot and spring upwards rapidly - as though it were contacting a very hot burner on a stove. The hips should remain level and virtually motionless throughout the exercise, with very little vertical displacement. After hopping for the indicated time on the left leg, switch to the right leg and repeat the exercise.

Why hop on one foot instead of bounding from foot to foot, as runners usually do during their drills? For one thing, it's very difficult to move fast while you are bounding, so bounding is not very much like sizzling through a 5-K or 10-K race. In contrast, you can move very quickly during the one-leg hops, so your power expands dramatically and your coordination during high-speed running improves greatly. Eventually you'll learn to move more quickly and efficiently. Research carried out by Russian scientists indicates that one-leg hopping is far superior to bounding at inducing improvements in leg speed ("Muscles and the Sprint," *Legkay Atletika*, # 5, pp. 8-11, 1992, cited in *Fitness and Sports Review International*, pp. 192-195, December 1992).

For similar reasons, the one-leg squat (exercise # 2) is superior to a very popular, traditional exercise - the two-legged squat. While a much greater load can be hoisted on the shoulders during a two-legged squat, that weight is distributed through two legs, not one, so the actual resistance per leg is often less. In addition, the trunk of the body is often inclined significantly forward in a two-legged squat but remains nearly vertical in a one-leg effort, so the latter more closely parallels the form required for running. Plus, for purposes of maintaining balance, the feet are often angled outward during the two-leg squat, which is unnatural to running, while the feet point straight ahead during a one-leg effort. Overall, the one-leg squat has the added advantage of being safer, since less total weight is used.

The third exercise - the high-bench step-up - is like climbing hills in the comfort of your own home or gym. You're basically lifting your body repeatedly against the force of gravity and powerizing your hamstrings, quads, and gluteals in the process. Like hill workouts, the step-up should improve your running economy and LT.

Overall, the three strength exercises carry little risk of injury, require just a small amount of your time, and are very specific to the actual act of running. The strength triad will improve both your coordination and leg-muscle power, and after several weeks you'll notice that your legs feel much stronger and that your stride length and frequency have improved. As your strength improves, please make the exercises more difficult by increasing the number of reps, adding additional sets of each exercise, and then increasing the total resistance by holding dumbbells in your hands (you can start with five-pound 'bells and work upward).

OWEN ANDERSON

CHAPTER 9

ADDITIONAL POINTS ABOUT LT:
THE ROLE OF TRAINING
VOLUME AND REST

Should you try to improve your LT by increasing your training volume? To put it another way, can running, cycling, or swimming more miles per week have a significant impact on LT? The answer is a qualified yes, because the effect of volume will be most pronounced in fairly unfit, non-experienced exercisers who are raising training volume significantly for the first time. Research carried out with previously sedentary lab rats found that rodents who ran for two hours per day increased mitochondrial enzymes much more than rats who scurried along for one hour daily (more mitochondrial enzymes usually mean a higher LT). In turn, the one-hour rats fared better than 30-minute per day trainees, which did better than rodents who hustled along for only 10 minutes per diem. The two-hour animals were also able to keep up a bristling treadmill pace for over twice as long as any of the other groups ("Skeletal Muscle Respiratory Capacity, Endurance, and Glycogen Utilization," *American Journal of Physiology,* vol. 228(4), pp. 1029-1033, 1975).

However, in experienced runners (both of the human and rat variety), increased mileage is much less likely to produce such striking effects on mitochondrial enzymes and LT. As we mentioned earlier, scientific research consistently shows that LT is best boosted by increases in intensity, rather than hikes in mileage. For example, scientists at the University Medical Hospitals in Freiburg and Ulm, Germany recently studied runners who either hoisted their training volume (mileage) by up to 100 percent over a four-week period or else lifted their average training speed while holding mileage steady. Training velocity was improved by replacing slow, moderately paced miles with 400-meter intervals at faster than 5-K pace, 1000-meter intervals at roughly 5-K speed, and "tempo running" at approximately 10-K pace ("Unaccustomed High-Mileage vs. Intensity Training-Related Changes in Performance and Serum Amino Acid Levels," *International Journal of Sports Medicine,* vol. 17(3), pp. 187-192, 1996). *After the four-week period, LT failed to improve at all in the increased-mileage runners - but soared by about 7 percent in the heightened-intensity group!* This upswing in LT was associated with improvements in performance of 5 to 17 percent.

Rest to Improve LT?

You can also aid your LT greatly by learning how

to *recover* from hard training in a strategic manner. In a study carried out at the University of Alberta in Canada, a group of well-conditioned athletes trained strenuously for six weeks and then cut back on training dramatically over a six-day period, resting completely for two of the six days, cutting normal workout duration by 67 percent on two other days, and slimming sessions by 33 percent on the other two days. This reduced-training group was compared with another group of athletes who simply kept on training at usual levels - and with a third group who did no training at all during the six days ("The Effects of a Reduced Exercise Duration Taper Program on Performance and Muscle Enzymes," *European Journal of Applied Physiology*, vol. 65, pp. 30-36, 1992).

Although LT was the same in all three groups at the end of the six-week training period (just before the six-day experimental period), there were major differences after the six days of rest or work were over. Basically, the reduced-training group lifted LT by slightly over 10 percent, the group which engaged in total rest failed to improve LT, and the group which continued to train hard actually experienced a deterioration of LT! There's an important lesson here: At least every six weeks (for some athletes it should be every three to four weeks), workouts should be reduced *significantly* for six or seven days to allow muscles to recover from strenuous training and create the new mitochondria, transporter proteins, and enzymes which will raise LT and also improve performance. It's also important to have at least one recovery day each week during which you do no training at all; these one-day furloughs give muscles a chance to "catch up" with their tasks of performing minor repairs and synthesizing increased quantities of necessary enzymes - and thus are good for increasing lactate threshold. Incessantly hard training can be the ruination of a quality LT.

CHAPTER 10

SPECIFIC LT WORKOUTS
AND AN OVERALL LT-LIFTING
PROGRAM FOR RUNNERS

An optimal seven-week period for enhancing LT (including six weeks of work and one week of rest) can proceed as follows (only the quality workouts are described; the rest of the weekly running would involve easy efforts; please note that the LT workouts progress in difficulty over the six-week training period):

Week 1

LT Session 1: Warm up, and then ramble for 20 minutes at a pace which is 10 to 12 seconds slower per mile than your current 10-K race tempo or 25 to 27 seconds slower per mile than your current 5-K race speed (these paces will be very close to your current LT velocity). Cool down with two easy miles.

LT Session 2: Warm up, and then run three to four one-mile intervals at your current 10-K pace (if you run only 5Ks and therefore don't have a current 10-K pace, this interval pace will be about 15 seconds per mile slower than your current 5-K tempo), with three-minute (jogging) recoveries in between. Cool down with two easy miles.

Week 2

LT Session 3: Warm up, and then perform the following activities in order:

> (1) Run 3/4 mile at your current 10-K pace
> (2) Do 50 ab crunches
> (3) Complete 5 chin-ups
> (4) Perform 15 push-ups
> (5) Complete 30 body-weight squats (fast)
> (6) Do 20 squat thrusts with jumps (burpees)
> (7) Run 3/4 mile at 10-K pace again
> (8) Perform 8 feet-elevated push-ups
> (9) Do 50 low-back extensions
> (10) Complete 15 bench dips
> (11) Do 15 squat and dumbbell presses with 10-pound dumbbells
> (12) Perform 20 lunges with each leg
> (13) Run 3/4 mile at 10-K pace again
> (14) Cool down with two miles of light jogging

VO2max Session 1: Warm up, and then run four to six 800s at your current 5-K pace, recovering after each work interval by jogging easily for the same amount of time it takes to complete the work interval. Finish the workout by cooling down with two easy miles.

LT Session 4: Run continuously over rolling terrain for one and one-half to two times the distance of your average daily run, working hard on all uphills, and maintaining an average pace which is about 30 to 45 seconds slower per mile than your current 10-K pace.

Week 3

LT Session 5: Warm up, and then run for two miles continuously at your current 10-K pace (please remember; if you only run 5Ks and don't have a current 10-K tempo, this will be about 15 seconds per mile slower than your current 5-K pace). Recover for five minutes, and then run two more miles at 10-K pace. Cool down with two miles of light ambling.

Economy Workout 1: Warm up, and then - on a hill which is roughly 200 meters from bottom to top - complete eight "reps", surging up the hill each time at what *feels* like 5-K race intensity (actual pace will be slower than 5-K striding because of the inclination). Recover by jogging back to the bottom, and finish the workout with 2 cool-down miles.

Week 4

LT Session 6: Warm up, and then ramble for 25 minutes at a pace which is 10 to 12 seconds slower per mile than your current 10-K tempo. Cool down with two easy miles.

VO2max Session 2: Warm up, and then run three to four one-mile intervals at current 5-K race pace, with five-minute jog recoveries in between work intervals and a two-mile cool-down at the end.

General Endurance Session 1: Run continuously for about two times the distance of your average daily run, maintaining an average pace which is about 45 seconds slower per mile than current 10-K pace.

Week 5

LT Session 7: Warm up, and then perform the following activities in order:

(1) Run 1/2 mile at your current 10-K pace
(2) Do 30 ab crunches
(3) Complete 4 chin-ups
(4) Perform 12 push-ups
(5) Complete 20 body-weight squats (fast)
(6) Do 15 squat thrusts with jumps (burpees)
(7) Run 1/2 mile at 10-K pace again
(8) Perform 7 feet-elevated push-ups
(9) Do 30 low-back extensions
(10) Complete 10 bench dips
(11) Do 10 squat and dumbbell presses with 10-pound dumbbells
(12) Perform 15 lunges with each leg
(13) Run 1/2 mile at 10-K pace again
(14) *Repeat steps 2-13 one more time (for two cir-*

cuits in all).

(15) Cool down with two miles of light jogging

LT Session 8 (The MCT1 Special): Warm up, and then complete eight two-minute intervals at close to maximal pace, with easy, four-minute jog recoveries in between. Stay relaxed and free-flowing during the two-minute work intervals; don't tighten up! Cool down with two easy miles at the end.

Week 6

LT Session 9: Warm up, and then complete four eight-minute intervals at your current 10-K pace, with only three minutes of recovery between intervals. Cool down with two miles of light jogging.

Economy Session 2: Please warm up, and then - on a very steep hill of 75 to 100 meters, complete 12 reps, surging up the hill each time at what *feels* like 5-K race intensity (actual speed will be slightly slower). Recover by jogging back to the bottom, and finish the workout with 2 miles of easy ambling.

LT Session 10: Run continuously (over rolling terrain, if possible) for one and one-half to two times the distance of your average daily run, working hard on all uphills, and maintaining an average pace which is about 30 to 45 seconds slower per mile than your current 10-K pace.

Week 7

Recovery: Cut mileage to 40 percent of normal levels (if you usually run 35 miles in a week, complete just 14), take an extra recovery day, and run easily all week, with one minor exception: About mid-week, warm up and then run eight 400s at 5-K pace, with one- to two-minute recoveries. This rest period will allow your body to "consolidate" the gains accruing from your six weeks of hard work, so that at the end of this seventh week, you'll have a stunning new LT!

That's it! In the first six weeks of this seven-week program, there are 10 LT workouts, two economy sessions, two VO2max efforts, and one general-endurance routine. There are enough workouts to propel your LT upward maximally - and an adequate number of efforts to *maintain* VO2max and economy. LT-type training can produce a true transformation in your running, but don't forget that it needs to be integrated well with other forms of work. For example, you should always build a good "base" of both mileage and strength before you undertake serious LT training; you can't simply plunge into heavy-duty LT exertions at the beginning of your training year.

If you would like to put LT training toward the beginning of your overall training cycle - ahead of VO2max, economy, and power development (and of course that's a decent idea, since LT gains will have the most profound impact on your running), you should first precede your LT-emphasis period with *at least* six weeks of both mileage expansion and general strength-building. For example, if your training year begins in January, as it does for many runners, you would want to gradually increase your mileage and build overall body strength (using the exercises listed in the circuits above or completing the circuits themselves) through at least mid-February before getting serious about LT and attempting to carry out the workouts outlined in the seven-week program. True, you could sprinkle a few LT sessions into your early "build-up", but you should wait to embark on the full LT program until you have a firm foundation of strength and endurance.

In addition, it's wise to devote just four to six weeks at a time to strenuous LT efforts, shifting over to other key training emphases (VO_2max, economy, or power) after your LT period is over. If you are cramped for time because of an impending race and can only reserve four weeks for LT, simply use the first four weeks of the above seven-week program (followed by a rest period of four to six days). Later in the year, when you return to LT training, you can pick up the last two weeks of hard workouts and then cycle back to the first four weeks, toughening the training sessions from the initial four weeks (by increasing the number of intervals, shortening the recoveries, and lengthening the continuous runs) as you do so. If you return to LT-building periods of training every 12 to 18 weeks or so, the most consistent thing about your running will be your steady improvement!

On average, if you improve your LT by 3 percent, your 10-K times will also improve by 3 percent. Raise LT by 10 percent - and your 10-K finishes will be 10-percent better. Lift LT by 20 percent - and you will truly shock your running acquaintances with your 20-percent upswing in 10-K speed *(Journal of Applied Physiology,* vol. 58(4), pp. 1281-1284, 1985). So - it's time to get started on your LT lift-off!

Of course, the above workouts represent only a small sample of the LT-lifting possibilities. For example, other "MCT1 Specials" would include:

(1) Running 45-second intervals at close to maximal pace, with two-minute recoveries,

(2) Completing 90-second intervals at close to maximal pace, with three-minute recoveries,

(3) Running "diagonals" on a soccer or football field, moving at close to top speed in a diagonal direction from a corner of one end zone to the far corner of the other end zone, jogging down the back line of the end zone, surging through the next diagonal, jogging along the back of the end zone, running another diagonal, and so on (start with 15 to 20 diagonals per workout and increase the number over time), and

(4) Running for a total of 60 minutes by alternating six-minute periods at marathon pace, which will be about 32 to 35 seconds per mile slower than 10-K velocity, with scalding two-minute blasts at 5-K race intensity. After each two-minute surge, be sure to return

quickly to the pace which is about 35 seconds slower per mile than 10-K velocity for the next six minutes, before returning to 5-K striding for two minutes; you're not allowed to jog slowly during this one! Note that you'll be beginning a 5-K-paced, two-minute interval every eight minutes - at six, 14, 22, 30, 38, 46, and 54 minutes into the workout (there are seven 5-K intervals in all). This is a very demanding workout, but it may seem paradoxical that it is included with the first three, since there is no maximal running involved and much work at marathon pace, which is below LT. However, the basis for the workout is that the ample lactate generated during the 5-K "blasts" is cleared and processed during the six-minute jaunts at marathon tempo, increasing lactate-clearance capacity.

Please note that with the exception of the diagonals session all of the above workouts can be completed in "cross-training" fashion on an exercise bicycle, if desired (for workout four, you'll just have to use your level of perceived exertion to guesstimate your marathon and 5-K intensities). Incidentally, all of the circuit sessions outlined earlier can also be completed on a bike rather than at the track; the idea is simply to attempt to match your perceived effort on the bike with the intensity you would feel while running at the indicated race pace. In case of bad weather (or sore legs), that's nice for runners to know!

It's important to note, too, that your current 10-K pace (or a tempo which is 15 seconds per mile slower than 5-K pace if you don't run 10Ks) is a particularly good workout intensity for LT improvement. Its special value is related to the fact that it is above LT speed - and therefore associated with fairly serious lactate production. Thus, it should stimulate muscles to increase their ability to clear and process lactate.

However, 10-K pace is not so far above LT that it must be confined to relatively short intervals. Whereas 5-K-paced intervals are seldom longer than 1600 meters, 10-K-speed intervals with durations of 2000, 2400, 2800, 3000, 3200, or even 4000 meters can be reasonably included in training sessions. These longer intervals can help you increase your ability to *sustain* quality paces for longer periods of time, in addition to hoisting your LT. Plus, practicing your current 10-K speed will no doubt increase your mental comfort at 10-K intensity, bolster your confidence, enhance your economy at 10-K pacing, and thereby increase the likelihood that you will be able to "step up" to faster speeds in future 10-K races.

Five of the workouts in the seven-week plan involve 10-K pace. Here are some additional LT-raising sessions which revolve around 10-K velocity (they progress in difficulty from number one through six):

(1) 6 X 1000 meters at current 10-K pace, with 150-second jog recoveries after the first five work intervals,

(2) 3 X 2000 meters at current 10-K pace, with three-minute jog recoveries after the first two work in-

tervals,

    (3) 3 X 2400 meters at 10-K speed, with three-minute jog recoveries,

    (4) 2 X 3000 meters, and then 1 X 2000 meters at 10-K velocity, with three-minute jog recoveries,

    (5) A 4000-, a 3000-, a 2000-, and then a 1000-meter interval at 10-K pace, with four minutes of rest after the 4000, three minutes after the 3000, and two minutes after the 2000, and

    (6) 4 X 2400 meters at 10-K speed, with two-minute jog recoveries in between intervals.

OWEN ANDERSON

CHAPTER 11

A VESTED INTEREST
IN LIFTING LT

As strange as it may seem, what you *wear* during your workouts can also have an impact on LT. Scientific research has shown that training in a weighted vest can help improve your lactate threshold.

Why would a vest make a difference to LT? Think of it this way: NASA researchers know that weightless space travel weakens leg muscles dramatically , because there is no gravitational resistance against which leg muscles must work. Daily muscular force production plummets significantly, and the weightless muscles "adapt" by getting smaller and weaker. The old adage "Use it or lose it" may be a bit trite, but it is also true.

In contrast, if you could spend a few days jumping around on Jupiter, the planet with the greatest gravitational force, you might transform yourself from the person with the weakest legs in the gym into a world-class slam-dunker. As gravitational force increases, the leg muscles are required to exert greater force to produce movment, and this spike in force production stimulates leg muscles to get considerably stronger.

Similarly, when you wear a weighted vest, your leg muscles are required to generate greater force to keep you moving along at a particular speed, since they must now transport a heavier weight. Over time, this increases leg-muscle strength, and improves LT. Once the legs are stronger, fewer muscle cells need to be recruited to maintain specific running speeds, and with a lower number of cells producing lactate, lactate levels drop.

We mentioned earlier in this book that an optimal strengthening program for runners must include exercises which are similar to the biomechanics of running. Running while attired in a weight vest is about as similar to running as you can get (after all, it is running). Along with hill repeats, vest work represents the ultimate form of strength training for runners.

Heikki Rusko is the man who has done most of the weight-vest investigating. He is an ingenious fellow (he's also the scientist who invented the "high-altitude house", a domicile which is at sea level but which internally contains an atmosphere similar to what prevails at about 10,000 feet of altitude; the beauty of Heikki's hut is that it produces all the performance-enhancing adaptations associated with high altitude but still allows athletes to carry out extremely high-quality training at sea level).

In Heikki's vest research, 12 experienced athletes wore vests during a four-week training block. Each vest tipped the scales at 10 percent of an athlete's total body weight, forcing leg muscles to work overtime during even routine activities like walking or standing. Athletes wore the vests throughout the day and during approximately three of their eight weekly workouts ("Metabolic Response of Endurance Athletes to Training with Added Load," *European Journal of Applied Physiology*, vol. 56, pp. 412-418, 1987).

Although the vests forced leg muscles to work harder than usual, the Finnish athletes were initially worse - not better - after the four weeks of vested training. The Finns needed about 3 percent more oxygen to run at 6:27 per mile pace (*e. g.,* running economy deteriorated), and their muscles also churned out more lactate at various running speeds (LT speed was lower). Overall, not a single positive benefit was present.

Fortunately, Rusko didn't give up. He asked the athletes to train and walk around for two more weeks without their beloved vests and then re-tested them. This time, the story was far different: Lactate threshold and VO2max each improved by 2 percent (compared to the beginning of the study), effects which would help the average endurance runner improve performances by approximately four percent. In addition, the athletes' abilities to sustain very high-speed running soared by 25 percent! And as if that weren't enough, the maximal velocity attained while running up stairs - a good indicator of leg-muscle power - increased by around 3 percent. In short, the four-week foray with weighted waistcoats gave the runners more "speed stamina" (because of their greater strength and higher LT) and made them more powerful, although a two-week recovery period was required before the positive effects appeared.

Why did these changes occur? Basically, the weighted vests increased force production by leg muscles but also probably changed the runners' basic running mechanics and muscular recruitment patterns slightly (to help support the greater weight). It's possible, too, that the vests may have activated "fast-twitch" muscle cells in the athletes' legs to a greater extent, compared to running without a vest (fast-twitch fibers tend to become active when force production increases). The temporary change in mechanics and recruitment undoubtedly produced the economy downturn. The same factors could have also soured LT a little, since less-trained muscle fibers might have been brought into play to support the extra weight (such fibers would be more likely to belch out lactate). If fast-twitch fibers indeed became more active during running because of the vest, you would naturally expect more lactate to be produced.

However, chronic vest-wearing would also force fast-twitch cells, which usually aren't very adept at using oxygen, to gradually and more fully develop their aerobic capabilities and diminish their lactate production. That would eventually (after a two-week rest period?) produce improvements in both lactate threshold and VO2max. In addition, slight changes in mechanics and recruitment would vanish once the vest stopped being worn. What would remain would be the improved specific strength for running, and this would heighten LT, as Rusko was able to observe.

The augmented specific strength also led to the major advance in power exhibited by the Finnish runners. When you've attained superior strength, all you have to do to boost your power is apply that strength more quickly.

To summarize Heikki's findings, it's clear that wearing a weighted vest *can* strengthen your leg muscles, lift LT, raise VO2max, and make you faster. The beneficial effects show up a couple of weeks after you *stop* wearing the vest, however, apparently because leg muscles need time to recover from the stresses of extra weight.

If you're considering the use of a weighted vest or some other weighted device, please bear in mind the following points:

It's probably a good idea to occasionally wear the vest throughout the day, as the Finnish athletes did. This produces a chronic overload on the leg muscles which can enhance strength.

Although vests have positive effects, "heavy hands" - weights carried in the hands as you run - won't improve your running. Although they fortify your shoulders and biceps, they won't do anything for your leg-muscle strength.

Attaching weights to your ankles is a bad idea. The extra poundage could be too stressful for your feet, ankles, shins, and knees and might wreck your running economy. Additional weight should be kept around the torso.

When should you include vest work in your training? The best time would no doubt be toward the end of a strength-training progression, e. g., after you have first gone through a fairly lengthy period of enhancing your whole-body strength and then running-related strength (for the latter, you would employ exercises which paralleled the mechanics of running). Combined with hill running, vest training would have a powerful effect on your LT and economy.

Of course, you wouldn't wear the vest during all of your workouts, nor would you wear the vest week after week throughout the rest of your year (or major cycle) of training. During the period of time during which you were emphasizing specific strength by employing hill work and vest running, two to three vest sessions per week would probably be about right (initially, you would not wear the vest while doing your hill repeats; that combination would come only after strength had improved appreciably). Extreme care must be taken, however: You can't simply load the vest chock-full of weight on your first workout and hope for the best. It's better to start with about three to four pounds of added resistance, and work slowly upward from there.

In the past, one of the key problems associated with vest training has been the ill fit of many of the vests (the darned things rattled around on your upper body and/or chafed your neck and shoulders). Fortunately, that difficulty is now resolved. A company called Training Zone Concepts produces a "Smart Vest™" which is both functional and fine-fitting. For information, give them a ring at 810-732-0849 (the toll-free number is 1-888-797-8378). There is no commercial affiliation between Training Zone Concepts and the author or publisher of this book.

CHAPTER 12

STRANGE BUT TRUE:
LT IMPROVEMENT IS GREAT
FOR THE 800-METER RUNNER,
AND 800-METER TRAINING IS
FINE FOR THE 5-K COMPETITOR

As we've already mentioned, lactate-threshold running velocity is a great predictor of performance prowess in endurance events like the 5K, 10K, half-marathon, and marathon. As LT speed rises, it simply "pushes" 5- and 10-K tempos to new heights and "pulls" half-marathon and marathon rambling upward - in the direction of new PRs.

However, although having a high LT velocity is critical for 10-K running and marathoning, there's no way that LT speed should be a big deal in 800-meter racing, right? After all, to run a super 800, you want real power - rippling leg muscles, high stride rates, lengthy strides, and tremendous tides of lactate flooding your muscles as they pour out the high-wattage anaerobic energy. In contrast, one aspect of building a great LT involves minimizing lactate production, the total opposite. Plus, the best techniques for heightening LT include running fairly long intervals at about 10-K pace and cruising through continuous, 25-minute tempo runs at a speed which is 10 to 15 seconds per mile slower than 10-K tempo. It's hard to understand why that sort of training would help you blast off like a rocket in an 800-meter competition.

However, that reasonable reasoning is dead wrong: LT speed is a great predictor of 800-meter prowess. As your LT velocity goes up, your 800-meter time improves dramatically. And as your 800-meter ability crests, so will your capacity to run a really fast 5K!

The Otago 800

You'll hear more about the connection between 800-meter and 5-K success in a moment. For now, here's the story behind LT velocity and your best-possible 800-metering: At the University of Otago in New Zealand, Gordon Sleivert and A. K. Reid recently evaluated 17 middle-distance runners (12 males and five females) of good ability ($VO_2max = 63.1$). The 17 athletes competed at 400, 800, 1500, and 5000 meters and were also checked for LT, VO_2max, and running economy (the three key physiological variables which best predict middle- and long-distance running success).

Well, we usually preach that aerobic development is fairly important for 800-meter performance (since about half of the energy needed for the race is generated aerobically), but guess what? Sleivert and Reid found that VO2max was totally unrelated to 800-meter times. In other words, runners with high VO2max values didn't run faster than those with low-ball figures. So much for the oxygen sermonizing!

800-meter times also didn't depend at all on running economy. If you're following along, that shouldn't be a surprise. We've already found out that being able to use oxygen at high rates (e.g., having a lofty VO2max) is no big deal for the 800. So why would we expect that being parsimonious with that common atmospheric gas should be a big deal, either?

But LT velocity? Since aerobic metabolism (either high, for VO2max, or low, for good economy) is no great shakes at prophesying 800 times, then "anaerobic" (oxygen-independent) energy creation must be the prime thing. And anaerobic metabolism means getting out there on the track and letting it rip, flooding the muscles with lots of lactate and creating all sorts of energy without utilizing much oxygen. On the other hand, having a high LT often means running fast without too much lactate. As we mentioned before, those are opposites, so how can LT be so important for 800-meter times?

Just the Facts

"If someone has a high LT velocity, then they can run faster with less lactate accumulation, compared to someone with a medium or low LT speed," says Dr.

Sleivert, who is a fine coach in addition to being a keen kinesiologist. Makes sense, doesn't it? But just in case it doesn't add up to you, let's use an extreme but edifying example: If someone has an LT velocity of 300 meters per minute, they can run an 800 in 2:40 (which is exactly 300-meter per minute pace) without getting the lactate waterfall going. On the other hand, someone with a lower LT speed of 250 meters per minute would produce huge dollops of lactate at 300-meter per minute pace and experience mega amounts of fatigue when trying to run the 800 in 2:40. The 300-LT person would be a much better 800-meter racer than the 250-LT competitor.

"To put it another way, remember that below LT speed your lactate level is pretty placid and constant while above LT your lactate level rises steadily and predictably as your running pace increases. That means that as your LT speed gets faster, you have more running speeds with calm lactates (those are all the ones which are below LT pace), and - most importantly - your running speed at any given lactate concentration is faster. As a result, you can run more quickly without excessive fatigue," observes the man from Otago (remember that running becomes steadily more difficult as blood-lactate levels advance; if these lactate advances can be arrested, then it becomes easier to run faster).

Here are some cool examples of that: Let's say that when you run the 800 in 2:00 (a nice thought!), your lactate concentration is 14 mmol/liter. However, you improve your LT speed so much that lactate only rises to 12 when you zip through 800 meters in 2 minutes. You can still tolerate a lactate level of 14, though, so - hey! - why not stoke up your running with a little more anaerobic energy, pushing lactate up to that magic 14 number? When you do, you'll zip through the race in just 1:55 or 1:56!

Or, let's say your LT speed is 300 meters per minute, which produces a lactate concentration of 4, and you run your 5Ks at 315 meters per minute, with a lactate level of 8.. However, by following the training dictates outlined in this book, you manage to raise your LT velocity to 315 meters per minute. Since your lactate is now a simpering 4 mmol/liter at 315 meters per minute, and you can tolerate 8 mmol in the 5K, you do the right thing: You shoot your 5K pace up to 330 meters per minute, giving you that nice lactate buzz of 8 mmol again, and improving your 5-K time by a not-too-shabby 43 seconds.

Well, we've got this LT speed and 800-meter racing connection down pat now, and the last example shows that it doesn't sound that much different from what we want to achieve in order knock off some great 5Ks and 10Ks. To put it simply, you become much better as a runner if you can move really fast without churning up the lactate waters too much (e. g., without producing mega-advances in blood lactate). That's true for the 800 - and for the 5K and 10K, too.

And that suggests that aerobic development is important after all in the 800 (otherwise, your muscles would spew out too much lactate). We're not contradicting what we said earlier here: The way to think about it is to realize that VO$_2$max is *not* an important predictor of 800-meter success when you look at a *group* of runners. After all, the high-VO$_2$max gal or guy might not be able to generate enough energy anaerobically to compete well in the two-lap race. She (or he) could be beaten easily by the mediocre O$_2$-max runner who could turn out a lot of energy oxygen-independently.

However, when we look at you as an *individual*, it's immediately clear that you *do* have to work on your VO$_2$max if you want to run your best 800. That's because upgrading your heart's thumping power and your leg-muscles' oxygen-grabbing capacity (the two components of VO$_2$max) is one way to keep you from generating too *much* lactate during the race.

And upraising your LT - getting really good at running fast without turning on the lactate spigot - will help you even more. It's just a question of knowing how - and when - to try to maximize LT speed.

Fortunately, the how part is easy: Key workouts for LT enhancement have already been outlined in this book. To answer the "when question," if you're training for 800 meters, you should do these kinds of workouts only after you've gone through at least a two-month period of "general running," which includes some long aerobic running, a few interval workouts at 5-K pace, and a generous portion of hill climbing. And do them before you begin to focus on 400-meter-type training for your 800s.

What's that? Well, we almost forgot to tell you that in addition to LT speed, 400-meter time is a tremendous predictor of 800-meter performance, too. After all, we can't let LT velocity stand around by itself and be lonely. You do need a great LT, but you also need to fully develop your anaerobic (400-meter) capacity if you want to run your best possible 800. LT and anaerobic capacity are the "twin towers" of 800-meter racing.

So, that means getting out on the track and doing some 200-meter intervals which are two seconds per 200 faster than current 800 race pace - and some 400-meter intervals which are three seconds per 400 faster than current 800 race pace. Such intervals will develop your speed and anaerobic capacity (recoveries from these intervals can last for several minutes; you should feel strong and ready to go before you begin a subsequent work interval).

To foster speed endurance (the ability to run fast while tired), you'd want to cover some 1000-meter intervals in which the first 800 is about 30 seconds or so slower than 800-meter race pace but the last 200 is at exact race pace, and also some 200-meter intervals at exact race pace, *with only 10 seconds of rest in between.* To optimize finishing power, it's also nice to run some repeat 300s. For these, the first 100 should be easy striding, but the last 200 should be at race speed. Recoveries shouldn't last for more than a minute or so.

Lactate Stacking

Sleivert himself likes to use the "Lactate Stacker," a red-hot workout which involves warming up and then alternating 40-second work intervals (at 400-meter race pace), with 20-second recoveries (jogging). It's appropriate to start with two sets of five to six repetitions of the 40-second surges, building up to two sets of 10 to 12 reps over the course of a six-week macrocycle. This session is great for developing anaerobic capacity - and the ability to tolerate acidic conditions inside your muscle cells (the kind of conditions which prevail near the end of an 800-meter race). Of course, it's good for LT, and - strangely enough - this workout isn't bad for good-ole' VO2max either, since it keeps heart rates at near maximum for the duration of each set.

Another gemstone training session for upraising anaerobic capacity, also recommended by Sleivert, is to warm up and then pile up 200-meter repeats at a pace which is two seconds per 200 faster than 800 tempo, with 30 to 45 seconds of recovery. Again, you can start with two sets of five to six reps, gradually increasing to 10 to 12 reps over time.

Whoa! Don't forget that while you're doing all that speedy stuff, you've got to maintain your VO2max and LT speed , too. Otherwise, you'll start bathing your leg muscles in a sea of lactate again - and bury your mind in a mountain of fatigue. A weekly VO2max or LT session, along with a weekly steady run of 45 minutes or so, should be helpful here.

Oh - there's one other thing we forgot to tell you: Sleivert found that 800-meter capability is a pretty good predictor of 5-K performance (runners with superior 800-meter times were also the ones with the best 5-K times, too). That's because doing some of the things which are necessary for 800-meter running, like giving VO2max an elevator ride, lifting LT, and developing higher footspeed, are all wonderful for 5-K racing, too. The bottom line is that even if you've never run an 800-meter race in your whole running career, conducting some workouts which are great for the 800 will also give your 5-K running new life!

OWEN ANDERSON

CHAPTER 13

IS A HEART MONITOR
USEFUL FOR LT TRAINING?
WHAT SHOULD YOU DO IF
YOU'RE A CYCLIST OR SWIMMER?

I f you have purchased a heart monitor and usually run your workouts or races at a particular heart rate (or a fixed percentage of your maximal heart rate), you've eliminated a big problem: You don't have to worry about estimating your actual running pace during your exertions or try to assess the overall quality of your effort by how you feel. You can let the monitor "be the judge."

Your effort - at least your cardiovascular effort - is precisely defined by the reading on the face of your heart-rate receiver. If you have an upscale monitor, any excessive deviation from your desired pulse triggers warning whoops from your device; with a low-end model, you need only to glance at your receiver every minute or so to find out if you're doing the right thing. You can cruise through your whole race or workout at the exact heart rate that you want, without worries about your actual running velocity.

Using a monitor can be pretty relaxing; during workouts, you can focus intently on your running form and how you feel, listen for the occasional communiques from your receiver, and just let the miles roll by as you run wherever you want to run. With a monitor, there's no need to be concerned about whether you're exceeding a level of cardiovascular effort which you know you can handle. However, in spite of this ease, precision, and comfort, if you use a monitor to measure the intensity of your workouts and races, you're probably headed for trouble.

The trouble will come in a variety of ways, but a key source of difficulty is something called "cardiac drift." This phrase simply refers to your heart's perverse tendency to avoid a constant rate of functioning. More specifically, cardiac drift means that your heart rate tends to rise slowly but steadily as you run, even when you're cruising along at a constant pace. And the magnitude of this drift is usually more than just a pesky beat or two: Heart rates can rise by as much as 20 beats per minute during runs lasting less than 30 minutes, even when those runs are conducted *at a constant velocity!*

There's no need to worry about *why* cardiac drift occurs, although staying well hydrated before and during your effort can partially control - but not eliminate - your heart's tendency to beat faster and faster (if your exertion is going to last for about 40 to 45 minutes or more and you're going to be sweating fairly profusely, you should try to thwart drift by drinking 10 ounces of fluid 10 minutes before you start and taking in five to six swallows of liquid every 15 minutes thereafter).

If you monitor your efforts by using heart rate, you *do* need to consider what effect drift will have on your running. Basically, if you're locked into a particular heart rate for a race or long workout, drift will force you to run slower and slower as the exertion proceeds, even though you *have the ability to maintain your even pace.* You might be cruising along fairly comfortably at seven-minute pace and a heart rate of 160, for example, until drift sends your ticker up to 166. If you're too in love with your heart rate, you would ease off on your pace until you simmer your cardiac center down to 160, and you would suddenly find yourself at 7:15 tempo, instead of the seven-minute effort *which you actually could handle.* In a race, that would leave you with a disappointing time; in a workout, you would spend less time practicing your goal pace - and therefore develop less efficiency at that pace. Most of the time, it's better to just let heart rate rise slowly and steadily during your effort (as long as you're still feeling OK). Let your pace and your level of fatigue - not the gadget on your wrist - be your guide to what you can do.

A Range of Paces

Of course, another difficulty associated with using a heart monitor is that a specific heart rate - the one a coach has recommended for a race or workouts, or the one you've decided to use based on a recommendation in a newsletter or running book - *is going to produce a variety of different running paces during your training.* We've already seen that this can happen because of cardiac drift, but another factor is that heart rate is quite sensitive to environmental conditions - and your psychological state. Generally, your heart rate is going to be higher than usual when the weather is hotter or more humid - and also when you're more tense and irritable than usual.

To see what can actually happen, let's say that you want to develop the ability to run a half-marathon at 90 percent of your max heart rate - a laudable goal. And let's say that - in deference to the specificity of training principle - you've decided to run many of your workouts at that specific intensity. That sounds good in theory!

The first time out, on a fairly hot and humid day, you run for an hour at your desired heart rate - 90 percent of maximal. Your average running pace for the whole workout turns out to be seven minutes per mile.

The next time you train at 90 percent, it's a perfect day for running - cool and dry. You zip along for an hour again at 90 percent of max, but when you get through, you discover a startling fact: Your pace was 6:45 per mile!

The third time out, it's hot and humid *and windy.* You're still stuck like glue on 90 percent of max heart rate, though, and so your hour passes at a comparatively lethargic pace of 7:20 per mile (remember that when it's hot and humid, heart rate rises more quickly than usual, bringing you to a specific rate at a slower running pace; running against wind compounds the problem).

On your fourth encounter with 90 percent of max heart rate, weather conditions are fine again, but you've just had a fight with your spouse. You're tense and excitable, sending your heart rate to higher-than-usual levels. So, you reach 90 percent of max too easily. In fact, at 90 percent, your running pace is only 7:30 per mile.

Suddenly it's race day, and you're pretty sure you can handle the half-marathon at 90 percent of max heart rate, no matter what. But when you finish the race, are people going to ask you, "Hey, what heart rate did you have out there?" Or will they ask you about your time? And are *you* going to care more about your heart rate or your actual finishing time?

Heart Versus Legs

The point is that if you have even an ounce of competitive spirit, you're going to be more concerned about your overall performance time than the rate at which your heart was pumping during the race. Paradoxically, though, you've been training to run the race with a particular heart rate - not in a particular time. You're at the mercy of your heart - and that expensive strap you've got around your chest!

Wouldn't it make more sense to choose a sensible goal *pace* for your half-marathon (say about 15 seconds slower per mile than 10K velocity), a pace which will bring you to the finish line in the time that you want, and then learn to handle that pace under a variety of different conditions during training? *Practicing that pace will give you the precise neuromuscular coordination and the precise leg-muscle functioning that you'll want on race day.* Who cares if your heart strays above some pre-defined rate of ticking? Believe me, your ticker will be none the worse for wear on the following day.

Basically, you have to make a decision about your training. You know that environmental conditions and your psychological state are going to vary on different workout days. Higher temperatures and humidity will send your heart rate up, as will tension and anxiety; cool weather and calmness will bring it down. You can stick with a specific heart rate - and therefore let actual running pace wander all over the map. Or you can stick with a specific pace - and let heart rate vary enormously. Which is better?

Obviously, sticking with a pace and letting heart rate vary is preferable. As mentioned, attaching yourself to a pace teaches your leg muscles and nervous system to function more effectively at that goal speed. The more you practice the pace, the better will be their coordination and efficiency - at that pace. The less you practice the pace, the lower will be coordination and economy.

In contrast, the heart's coordination and economy do not vary. The heart doesn't need to practice beating away at 90 percent of maximal to get good at it; it already has that down-pat. It's just as efficient at 90 percent of max as it is at 87 percent of max - or at 93 percent.

Basically, your heart is pretty much along for the ride. It will do what your leg muscles tell it to do (within limits, of course; the legs can't tell the heart to beat faster than max heart rate, for example). If your heart's been whacking away at 93 percent of max for a good deal of time, it will never shout down to the leg muscles, "Hey fellas! This has been going on long enough. I'm getting tired, so will you slow down please?"

The truth is that your legs become fatigued far more quickly than your heart. The heart slows down when the leg muscles slow down, not the other way around. That's why the *focus* of your training should be on your leg muscles - that is, on the pace created by the leg muscles. Your goal should be to develop greater fatigue resistance in those leg muscles at your desired paces. You don't have to worry about the heart getting fatigued: That old fellow can pound away at high rates for long periods of time. Your leg muscles are your weak link.

And yet training based on heart rate makes the heart dominant and the leg muscles subordinate - just the opposite of what should occur! If you really want to run a race at a goal pace, practice that pace, not a heart rate. You can let your heart rates roll around a bit.

Always remember that your heart is an imperfect indicator of what's happening to your leg muscles. An increase in heart rate *might* indicate increased stress in your leg muscles, or it might just represent tension, drift, or the fact that a little more blood has moved toward your skin for cooling on a hot day. Don't enshrine an imperfect indicator as the absolute dictator of your training and racing.

What is Your Lactate-Threshold Heart Rate?

There's an incredible amount of information floating around about how to train with a heart monitor, but - unfortunately - a lot of it is worthless. For example, you might read or hear that the best training intensity for raising lactate threshold - the key indicator of performance - is 82 to 88 percent of max heart rate. If someone tells you that, you've learned something very important: You should be very suspicious of what they tell you about endurance training.

That's because there's absolutely no scientific

evidence that this is true. In fact, the available research says that for runners, moving along at 10-K pace (which often coincides with around 90 to 93 percent of max heart rate) is a more time-efficient way to boost threshold and produces larger increases in LT. Second, while it's true that training at your threshold can probably raise it pretty well, too (that's why tempo runs are so darned good), threshold heart rate varies considerably between individuals. For example, in some people threshold occurs at 65 percent of max heart rate. In others, it's at 75 percent. Experienced, competitive endurance athletes often check in at 85 to 88 percent (but it may be as low as 80 or as high as 90), and some of the elite Kenyan runners don't reach threshold until they get to 92 to 94 percent of max.

The bottom line? To lift LT if you're a runner, you're better off forgetting about heart rate and training at well-defined running paces. Things get a little more complicated if you're a cyclist, however. For one thing, a particular speed can be attained with a variety of different gear ratios on the bike. Each gear ratio will have a specific impact on muscle recruitment patterns and muscular force production, both of which will influence lactate production. Thus, a particular speed may represent LT in one gear - but may actually be above or below LT using a different gear combination. In addition, bicycle races tend to feature long, steep hills to a much greater extent, compared to running races. In fact, most quality bike races aren't considered true races unless at least a few severe hills are part of the course; in contrast, many running courses are pancake flat, because race directors and runners themselves are highly attracted to "PR" courses (routes on which the chances of setting a personal record are enhanced). Of course, once you throw in the effect of inclination, estimating whether or not you are at LT (or 2.5 percent above it) becomes extremely difficult to do. Basically, LT will be reached at slower cycling speeds on hills, but the exact LT point is almost impossible to determine.

For those reasons, I often recommend that cyclists use heart rate to carry out their LT training, in spite of all the pitfalls associated with heart-rate monitoring. Fortunately, by focusing on some fairly high intensities (heart rates), it is possible to conduct some decent LT training on the bike.

First, though, you need to be absolutely certain that you know your true maximal heart rate. The popular 220-minus-age formula is a disaster; it simply predicts an average heart rate for a population of similar-aged people, and the standard deviation is quite large (a little over 12 beats per minute). This basically means that for a population of 50-year-old athletes, for example, even though 220 minus age predicts a max heart rate of 170, the basic "spread" of max heart rates, accounting for approximately 95 percent of all individuals aged 50, will actually range between 145 and 195. Worse yet, 2.5 percent of 50-year-olds will have max heart rates greater than 195, and 2.5 percent will be lower than 145, even though 170 is supposedly max heart rate in this group. If a 50-year-old athlete who believes his max heart rate is 170 but has a true max of 150 attempts to LT-train at

90 percent of max (90% X 170 = 153), he will actually be attempting to train above his maximum! At the other end of the spectrum, someone with a true max of 190 who trains at 90% X 170 will end up at only 153/190 or 80 percent of maximum - too low to give LT a real shove upward.

It's important to note, too, that if you're a runner who wants to carry out some LT training on the bike, you should be aware that your max cycling heart rate will often be eight to 12 beats per minute lower on the bike, compared to running. While that may seem strange, it's once again a sign that the heart follows what the muscles are doing, not the other way around. If your max heart rate while running is 178, it may be only 168 while cycling, and a 90-percent workout would center on a heart rate of 90% X 168, not 90% X 178.

If you want to actually reckon your max heart rate on the bike, it's easy: Simply warm up with 10 to 15 minutes of easy pedaling, and then ride "full-blast" at nearly maximal power output (while maintaining an optimal rpm of 90 to 95 or so) for two minutes. Pedal very, very easily against little resistance for 60 to 75 seconds, and then work at maximal capacity again for two more minutes. Your heart rate should almost "top out" after this second two-minute surge (Make sure you get permission from your primary-care physician before you try this, however).

Some decent LT-raising bike workouts would then be:

(1) 8 X 4 minutes at 95 percent of true maximal heart rate, with three-minute recoveries between work intervals (4 minutes at 95 percent of max heart rate actually means that after two minutes your heart rate should rise to about 95 percent - and stay there for the remainder of the interval; remember that it always takes the heart a little while to "catch up" with the leg muscles),

(2) 4 X 10 minutes at 90 percent of maximal heart rate, with four-minute recoveries between work intervals (again, give the heart the first two minutes of the interval to get up to 90 percent),

(3) 30 to 40 minutes of continuous riding at 85 to 87 percent of max,

(4) Two hours of continuous riding, with five-minute surges going up to 90 to 95 percent of max every 15 minutes (e. g., at 15, 30, 45, 60, 75, 90, and 105 minutes into the workout), and

(5) "MCT1" specials incorporating 45- to 120-second blasts at close to maximal intensity, with two- to four-minute recoveries (there's no need to worry about actual heart rate here).

Swimmers can give their LTs huge lift-offs by using exactly the same workouts (simply substitute "stroking" for "riding" in the above descriptions). Some coaches, especially swimming coaches, get really high-tech and measure heart rates at various blood-lactate levels. They then define workouts as "easy" or "aero-bic" if they are at a heart rate below the rate which produces a lactate concentration of 2 mmol/l, and they say that "threshold" workouts are *at* the heart rate which lifts lactate to 4 mmol/l, while "hard" efforts are at heart rates associated with lactate above 4 mmol. The task then is to merely find the right balance of easy, threshold, and hard efforts.

That coaching philosophy is great, except for a couple of things. First, if training is going well, the paces associated with 2 and 4 mmol/ of lactate will increase steadily over time, so finger pricking for lactate detection will have to take place on a regular basis.

However, the bigger problem is that threshold doesn't always occur at 4 mmol/l. Some athletes reach threshold at 2 mmol, while others don't hit it until they get up to 7. For those individuals who reach threshold at 2, a workout *at* 2 will no longer be an easy session; for those who attain threshold at 7, training at 4 will be far too light for optimal LT advancement.

OWEN ANDERSON

CHAPTER 14

CAN A LACTATE MONITOR
HELP YOU "STICK" TO YOUR LT?

Knowing your blood-lactate concentrations during training can help you in a number of ways, but there has traditionally been a big problem with reckoning lactates during workouts: The needed equipment has been very expensive - and much too cumbersome to drag to the track or cross country course for a training session. In addition, most of us don't have easy access to an exercise physiology laboratory equipped with lactate-measuring equipment, so we can usually only guess how much lactate is simmering in our bloodstreams when we do "tempo" workouts or hurry through intervals on the track.

Until now. A company called Sports Resource Group, Inc. is distributing a convenient little device - the Accusport™ Portable Lactate Analyzer - which is small enough to hold in the palm of your hand and cheap enough so that you won't have to take out a second mortgage on your home if you want it. Best of all, the little thing is darned accurate, giving readings almost identical to those obtained using heavy-duty, upper-price-bracket lab equipment.

Recently, scientists at Ithaca College in New York put the little monitor through its paces. 31 well-trained cyclists (16 males and 15 females) ranging in age from 16 to 43 years exercised at different intensities while their blood lactates were checked by both the Accusport™ and a "big boy" - the YSI Model 1500, which is a standard piece of equipment in many university exercise labs.

The Accusports™ (two were used in the study) fared extremely well. For example, when the subjects were at rest, the YSI gave lactate readings of about 1.17, while the Accusports™ checked in at 1.24 and 1.44. At 70% VO2max, the "ole' reliable" YSI settled at 2.14, while the Accusports cozed up just a tiny notch to 2.24 and 2.26. During a nearly maximal test which pushed the YSI needle to 13.21, the Accusports™ were not far away at 13.16 and 13.95. And during a Wingate Test of Anaerobic Capacity, the YSI hung in at around 14.52, while the Accusports™ were only a tick or two away at 14.66 and 14.86. Such readings are so close to the YSI "gold standard" that the only conclusion to draw is that the Accusport™ can be used confidently and successfully by athletes during workouts.

Good enough so far, but that still leaves us with two key questions. How would you use the

Accusport™ if you actually bought one? Could the pocket-sized device actually help make you a better runner, cyclist, or swimmer?

The answer to the latter question is definitely yes, although you have to remember that the Accusport™ is not a magical contraption which will automatically make your training better - and your performances higher. You do have to use the appliance wisely.

Putting the Little Accusport™ to Use

One application immediately became apparent at a recent meeting of the American College of Sports Medicine (the same venue at which the news about Accusport™ reliability was announced). In a paper presented at the meeting, researchers from the University Estacio de Sa and the University Gama Filha in Brazil used lactate measurements to accurately predict 5-K performances.

In this Brazilian study, 28 middle- and long-distance runners ran for five-minute intervals at various speeds on the track until they were able to find a speed (in meters per minute) which produced a blood-lactate reading of 4 millimoles per liter (when blood was withdrawn 30 seconds after the end of a five-minute interval). All 28 athletes also participated in a 5-K race.

The Brazilian scientists unearthed a very interesting relationship: Once the running speed which produced a lactate concentration of 4 millimoles/liter was identified, it was very easy to predict 5-K race velocity. In fact, all one needed to do was add about 14 meters per minute to the speed which caused lactate to ascend to 4. In practical terms, here's how this relationship might work for you: After running at various velocities during 5-minute intervals, you find - after a fair amount of finger pricking - that running at six-minute mile pace (268 meters per minute) gives you a blood lactate of about 4 mmol/liter. That being true, your predicted 5-K pace is 268 + 14 = 282 meters per minute, or 5:42 per mile. If you haven't run a 5K in a long time, or if you've only run 5Ks under pretty horrid environmental conditions which don't give you a true picture of your 5-K ability, that can be a pretty useful pace to know about.

For one thing, predicting your 5-K pace leaves you room for a pretty nifty workout. Using the example from the preceding paragraph, you could run some 1200s at 282-meter per minute tempo, which would mean completing each 1200 in 1200/282 = 4.25 minutes (that is, 4 minutes and 15 seconds). Another nice thing to do would be to work on your LT for six weeks (a six-week macrocycle) and then re-test yourself to see which running speed coincided with 4 mmol/liter of lactate. If you've done the right thing, your LT speed should be higher, which would also mean that your 4 mmol/liter speed would also be faster. If your Accusport™ tells you that your 4 mmol/liter pace is indeed a nicer number, you'll have confidence that your training is progressing as expected.

Other Applications

We shouldn't forget that there are other ways to employ the Accusport™, too. For example, you can check your lactate after your fairly intense workouts. If these are sessions which you repeat on a regular basis during your training year, you'll be able to obtain some valuable information. For example, suppose you like to carry out 2000-meter intervals at about your 10-K race pace, and you do this every two weeks or so. If you take your lactate level at the end of the last interval, and do this after every such workout, a declining lactate level over time will show you that your fitness is indeed improving.

You could also graph your lactate production at various running paces in order to chart your LT-lifting progress. The easiest way to do this is to run five-minute intervals at a pace which is, in order, 30 seconds slower per mile than 10-K tempo, 15 seconds slower per mile, *at* 10-K speed, 15 seconds faster, and 30 seconds faster per mile than 10-K pacing. For example, if you run the 10K at about six minutes per mile, you could conduct a workout in which you warm up, run for five minutes at 6:30 per mile pace, five minutes at 6:15 tempo, five minutes at 6:00, five minutes at 5:45, and finally five minutes at 5:30, or 30 seconds per mile faster than 10-K alacrity. In each case, you would recover for just two *or* three minutes between work intervals (choose one; don't vary it), and during the recovery you would check your blood lactate as soon as possible after the work interval ended. Each lactate reading would then be marked on graph paper in line with its corresponding pace. If this workout is then repeated after four to six weeks of solid LT training, the line connecting the lactate points should be lower (e. g., almost every speed utilized during the workout should correspond with a lower lactate reading).

Cyclists can do something quite similar on their exercise bikes. For example, a lactate-charting workout could involve warming up and then riding at 180, 210, 240, 260, 280, 300, and 320 Watts for six minutes each, with two or three minutes of recovery between intervals and the lactate test performed as soon as possible after each work interval ends. Again, the sign of LT progress would be a lowering of lactate concentrations at the various power outputs during subsequent tests.

And of course, you can use the Accusport™ to try to locate your real LT speed. However, be aware that this will require a lot of finger sticking, since you'll actually have to graphically plot your lactate concentration at a pretty wide range of running speeds (each of which will require a poke) in order to find the velocity at which lactate levels start to really climb. Be aware, too, that choosing an LT velocity from such a graph is not necessarily a precise endeavor, so much so that if you're a runner, you may be better off just sticking with 12 seconds slower per mile than 10-K pace as your guesstimate of LT velocity. Also, as we've mentioned over and over again, you should know that scientific research supports the idea that training at exactly 10-K pace, which is slightly faster than LT speed, is actually *better* for raising LT than training at LT itself, and of course you can identify your 10-K pace without using the Accusport™ at all. The bottom line is that you can run 10Ks fairly regularly and use your race pace for LT-enhancing workouts, instead of navigating through the ins and outs of blood-lactate measurement.

Mistakes

And one thing you'll definitely want to avoid is the popular practice of "lactate-zone" training, or LZT. In this form of training, you may attempt to carry out a certain percentage of your running or cycling below a lactate level of 2 mmol/liter, another percentage between 2 and 4 mmol, another fraction between 4 and 8, and yet another percentage above 8 (the percentages and actual lactate numbers vary from lactate guru to guru). Please remember that there's *no scientific research at all to support this form of training,* even though it certainly sounds and looks scientific when it is presented in book or article form. There is absolutely no way at all for the endurance athlete to know what percentage of training should be carried out within a particular range of lactate readings, nor is there even a way to identify the optimal lactate zones!

You also should be aware that the readings on the Accusport™ are good - but not absolute. In other words, the Accusport™ readings will vary around your true lactate level. This is not a big problem, though, and it certainly doesn't mean that the Accusport™ is not a useful device. What it does mean is that if your lactate level is 8.5 after a particular workout, and 8.7 after the same workout a few weeks later, that does not really foretell that your fitness has declined; the change may actually represent nothing more than the small, random errors made by the Accusport™ as it tries to gauge your true lactate level. Such small mistakes of a few tenths of a point are normal and are to be expected, so what you really need to look for are bigger moves.

For example, if your lactate is 8.5 when you run at a particular pace or conduct a specific workout and 7.5 four weeks later when you do the same kind of running, you can be very confident that you've raised your LTRV. Basically, reliability testing of the Accusport™ suggests that you should view lactate changes as real if they exceed about .5 mmol/liter. This means that if your lactate has been consistently at 6 mmol/liter when you run at six-minute per mile pace but suddenly changes to 5.6, you shouldn't be very confident that that's a real change. If it goes to 5.4, on the other hand, you can trust your little Accusport's contention that you've actually improved. Once you're at 5.4, though, don't get too happy until you reach 4.9 or lower - or too sad unless your lactate soars above 5.9.

However, you should be also be aware that diet, fatigue, recent training, and dehydration can all impact lactate readings. For example, a sudden increase in carbohydrate intake can boost lactate levels, without any changes in your basic fitness (that's why if you're going to take lactate readings on different days, you should always "standardize" your food intake on those days). Being more tired than usual or being somewhat dehydrated can also lift lactate levels unnecessarily high. As we mentioned earlier, the Accusport™ is not foolproof. It can be a valuable addition to your training but should not be relied upon as a *perfect* indicator of your fitness. As always, the true test of how good you are is competition.

How much does the diminutive Accusport™ cost? About $500 will bring the little beauty into your own home, along with some lactate test strips, control solutions, a personal lancet device (ouch!), some lancets, a carrying case, a fanny pack to keep the monitor with you as you run, and software and a connection cable to link your Accusport™ with your PC. The Accusport™ has a number of nice features: It can remember up to 101 previous lactate readings, which is very important for the individual who's forgetful about recording data. In addition, the batteries last for over 1000 tests, and it doesn't take the Accusport™ long to compute your lactate once a droplet of blood is inserted. Of course, the cost will certainly be too steep for the average jogger, but not too heart-stopping for the technically oriented athlete or coach who wants to utilize some of the training techniques described above. If you want to order, contact the Sports Resource Group at 914-747-8572 (the toll-free number is 1-888-474-5239). SRG also has an interesting web site at www.lactate.com

CHAPTER 15

SOME FINAL WORDS
ABOUT IMPROVING LT

One key aspect of training that most endurance athletes don't understand is that anything which improves economy (efficiency) will also tend to improve LT. That's because enhanced economy means lower energy utilization, and therefore a general drop in lactate production. As a result, the techniques traditionally used to optimize economy, including strength training and hill repeats, tend to be also good for LT-lifting. Detailed information about enhancing economy will be presented in a forthcoming book.

If you like the information presented in this book, then you will also like *Running Research News*, a newsletter which is published 10 times a year. *Running Research News* keeps you up-to-date on the latest information about endurance training, sports nutrition, strength training for endurance athletes, injury prevention, and sports medicine. Subscriptions are only $35 per year (checks, MasterCard, and Visa are accepted). Please mail your subscription payment to *Running Research News,* P. O. Box 27041, Lansing, MI 48909 USA. You may also fax your credit-card information to 517-371-4447 or call the newsletter at 517-371-4897 to place your order.

ABOUT THE AUTHOR

Owen Anderson, Ph.D., is the editor of *Running Research News*, a technical editor and monthly columnist for *Runner's World* magazine in the USA, the U.S. editor of the British newsletter *Peak Performance*, a regular contributor to the British edition of *Runner's World*, as well as *Men's Health, Walking,* and *Shape* magazines in the United States, and a frequent contributor to publications in Finland, Germany, the Netherlands, South Africa, and Sweden. He speaks frequently at seminars, coaches' clinics, sports-medicine conferences, race expos, and running camps throughout the United States, and he has coached and managed a number of elite runners.

Owen earned a B.S. in Zoology from the University of Rhode Island, where he was named the most outstanding undergraduate student in 1976 After receiving a Ph.D. from Michigan State University in 1983, he began carrying out research at MSU and published the first issue of *Running Research News* in 1985. Owen travels around the world to attend scientific conferences and interview outstanding exercise physiologists, coaches, and runners. He has made five trips to East Africa to study Kenyan runners and is currently working on a series of books about endurance training and sports nutrition. He lives in Lansing, Michigan with his partner and two daughters.